The Che... th

Edited by
Siobhán Cleary
In association with

TOWN
HOUSE

Published in 1993 by
Town House and Country House
42 Morehampton Road
Donnybrook
Dublin 4
Ireland
in association with RTE

A CIP catalogue record for this book is available from the British
Library.

ISBN: 0-948524-83-9

Cover design by Jack Hayden Design and Art
Cover photo of Siobhán Cleary by Frank Fennell Photography
Typeset by Printset and Design Ltd, Dublin
Printed in Ireland by Colour Books Ltd, Dublin

CONTENTS

Foreword: *Mary Raftery* v

Introduction: *Siobhán Cleary* 7

Alcohol: *Professor Anthony Clare* 9

Allergies: *Dr Paul Carson* 23

Arthritis and Rheumatism: *Dr Oliver FitzGerald* 35

Back Pain: *Mr Frank Dowling/Marie Elaine Grant* 45

Bereavement: *Thérèse Brady* 61

Bowel Problems: *Professor William Kirwan* 77

Breast Cancer: *Professor Niall O'Higgins* 87

Coughs and Wheezes: *Professor M X FitzGerald* 99

Depressive Illness: *Professor Patricia Casey* 109

Growing Old: *Professor Davis Coakley* 119

Heart Disease: *Professor Ian Graham* 131

Indigestion and Ulcers: *Professor Colm O'Moráin/
Dr Joan Gilvarry* 145

Infertility: *Professor Robert Harrison and his team at RCSI
and the Rotunda Hospital* 153

Men's Problems: *Mr T E D McDermott* 165

The Menopause: *Dr Máire Milner* 173

Mouth and Teeth: *Professor D B Shanley* 181

Pain: *Professor C A O'Boyle* 195

Premenstrual Syndrome: *Dr Valerie Donnelly* 207

Sexual Difficulties: *Mary O'Conor* 219

Sexually Transmitted Diseases: *Dr Fiona Mulcahy* 229

Skin Disorders: *Dr Sarah Rogers* 239

Sleep: *Dr Michael Buckley* 255

Smoking: *Carmel Buttimer* 269

Weight Control: *Mary Moloney* 283

Appendix: Incidence of Breast Cancer 294

Recommended Reading 295

Index 297

Siobhán Cleary has a background in theatre and teaching. She began her career as a journalist writing newspaper features and reporting on the *Gay Byrne Show*. She has been presenter of *Check Up* since it began, and she also produces educational videos for medicine and dentistry. She lectures in communication skills at the School of Dental Science, Trinity College, Dublin, and is married with two teenage children.

FOREWORD

Check Up is in its sixth year and is now firmly established as one of the most successful of RTE's information-based programmes. Its enormous popularity is due in the main to its concentration on the feelings and experiences of ordinary people who have had the misfortune at some stage in their lives to become patients.

Hundreds of these patients have featured on *Check Up* over the years, and we owe a great debt of gratitude to each and every one of them for allowing us into their homes and their lives. Everyone who has worked on the programme has been most impressed by how much private pain and anguish people are prepared to reveal, and by the fact that their motivation is always to help others to cope with similar problems.

It is equally the case that without the wholehearted co-operation of the medical profession in Ireland, *Check Up* would not have been able to provide the level of information and sound advice to the public that has now become its trademark. For all their support and help, we owe them our deep thanks.

Finally, there are those whose role within the programme has been central to its success. Anne McCabe founded the programme and was series producer for many years. She was responsible for setting the style and content of the programme, which has proved so popular with the public.

Ciana Campbell was co-presenter with Siobhán Cleary of *Check Up* for several years, and their high degree of professionalism and empathy contributed enormously to the credibility of the programme with both the public and the professionals alike.

Grateful thanks are due also to all the staff of RTE who have worked on the programme over the years, for their dedication and their commitment.

Mary Raftery
Series Producer
Check Up

THE CHECK UP TEAM 1993/94

Presenter:	Siobhán Cleary
Reporters:	Mary O'Sullivan, John Murray
Researcher:	Valerie Kennedy
Production assistants:	Una McHenry, Hilary Courteney
Producers:	Roy Esmonde, Karen Edmonds
Series producer:	Mary Raftery

INTRODUCTION

There was a time, not so long ago, when doctors were expected to know all the answers, and have a prescription for every ailment. Patients were supposed to do what they were told, and either get better or stop complaining. Thankfully all that has changed. We are now much better informed about medical matters, and realise that for the most part good health is up to us.

Over the last five years *Check Up* has played its part in bringing this change about. Our aim has always been to demystify medicine and make medical subjects more understandable to the lay person. We look for experts who will co-operate with us in explaining difficult ideas in a simple way and offer practical advice about treatment and living with different conditions. This book has the same purpose. Many of the authors are regular contributors to *Check Up*.

This is the first Irish health book of its kind. The list of authors reads like a Who's Who of Irish medicine, and many of the contributors have international reputations in their particular fields of expertise.

In drawing up the list of subjects to be covered, I decided to include some of the topics that created that greatest interest when they were featured on the programme, and some that we hope to do in the current series. Others have been included because they are more suited to a book than to a television programme.

I would like to thank all the distinguished writers who were involved, for their enthusiastic response to the idea of a *Check Up Guide to Good Health*, for taking so much time and care in the writing, and for allowing me the freedom to edit their material in order to make it more accessible to the reader.

Thank you to my publisher Treasa Coady for her guidance throughout the project, and to my assistant Keelin Shanley. I am particularly grateful to my children Susanna and Ronan who were the most enormous help whenever the computer threatened to turn nasty. A very special thanks to Joe for his constant love, support and encouragement.

Siobhán Cleary

ALCOHOL

PROFESSOR ANTHONY CLARE

What's the difference between an alcoholic and a heavy drinker? Would you know if someone close to you had a drink problem? Are you drinking too much? How accurate is the image of the drunken Irish? These are just some of the questions that are frequently asked about alcohol, its use and its abuse.

Psychiatrist Anthony Clare outlines the latest thinking on alcohol-related problems and describes the modern approach to the treatment of alcohol dependency . . .

ALCOHOL ABUSE

Advice concerning the health aspects of alcohol is simple. Consumed in modest quantities, alcohol poses no problems for psychological or physical health. In this area as in so many others, moderation is the best policy. In the light of evidence from research carried out over the past thirty years, it is now possible to talk in terms of 'safe' drinking and to advise the general public about how they may use alcohol sensibly and avoid its anti-social and harmful effects.

Alcohol is widely used in Irish society to mark life's passages – birth, marriage, childbirth, death. It permeates our social structures and activities – family relationships, the professions, political life, the arts, sport. It is a social lubricant, a psychological pick-me-up, helping us forget what we do not wish to remember, anaesthetising our pains, melting our guilts, banishing our remorse – in the short term, at least. But there is a price for all of these effects.

What must not be forgotten is that alcohol is a drug. It has widespread effects on the major organs of the body – liver, stomach, pancreas, blood, nerves, muscles and bones – most particularly on the brain itself. It is a depressant drug, not a stimulant, and its depressant effects go beyond reducing social unease and anxiety to release more basic, often aggressive and socially disruptive behaviour. There is a remorselessness about alcohol in the way that it exacts a price for its misuse in terms of physical ill-health, psychological disorder and social disruption.

ALCOHOL AND THE IRISH

The stereotype of the drunken Irish can be traced back to the medicinal use of alcohol in the cholera epidemics of the mid nineteenth century. Independent of the destructive effects of alcohol on cholera sufferers, the general public began to drink spirits in large amounts – over 16,000 poteen stills, for example, were discovered in 1833-4. The Temperance Movement, which began in the early nineteenth century in Skibbereen and New Ross, spread quickly and became a national movement under the leadership of Father Mathew. Throughout the first half of the twentieth century, Father Cullen's Pioneer Total Abstinence Association emphasised the spiritual and physical benefits to be derived from avoiding alcohol altogether – a policy that, implicitly at any rate, appeared to confirm that the Irish exhibited harmful tendencies when it came to drinking. This image received further confirmation from the public and damaging consequences of the over-indulgence in alcohol by many leading Irish artists including Brendan Behan and Flann O'Brien, and the portrayal of Irish alcohol use by writers such as Eugene O'Nell, Seán O'Casey and James Joyce.

This stereotype needs qualification, however. Ireland's alcohol consumption per head of population is the second lowest in Europe. The average Irish person drinks approximately eleven litres of absolute alcohol per year, whereas the average citizen of France, Germany, Spain and Luxembourg drinks over twenty litres in a year. A substantial proportion of our adult population – between 15 and 20 per cent – hardly drinks at all, a very much larger segment of the population than in other European countries or the US. We have low rates of physical diseases associated with alcohol abuse, such as liver cirrhosis or pancreatitis. On the other hand, the proportion of our disposable personal income spent on alcohol – 11.6 per cent – is among the highest in the world, substantially higher than the US (3.6 per cent) and the UK (6.5 per cent). This fact, in the words of psychiatrist Marcus Webb, 'cannot be good news, in particular, for the families of the many Irish who live below the poverty line'. Our psychiatric hospital admission rates for alcohol-related mental disorders are likewise high and community surveys suggest that the consumption of alcohol exacts a considerable toll in terms of marital and family disharmony and violence.

The answer to this paradox – low per capita consumption yet high rates of admission and psychiatric and social problems – may lie not so much in the amount of alcohol we consume but the way in which we consume it. French, Italian and other European patterns of drinking involve a steady, even daily, consumption of alcohol along with food, in communal settings such as the home, which is linked with the physical enjoyment of the taste and fragrance of alcohol. This type of consumption is not without its own problems, but these in the main are associated with the long-term effects of steady alcohol consumption on the digestive and related systems of the body. Irish drinking is characterised by a pattern of so-called 'binge drinking' in which the person goes for periods, often quite lengthy, with hardly any alcohol at all, then engages in episodes of exceptionally heavy drinking which are in turn followed by further periods of sobriety. There may be guilt and remorse concerning the binge and eventually further drinking may occur in an effort to relieve such feelings, leading to the typical cycle – periods of heavy drinking followed by periods of abstinence.

In further contrast to other patterns of drinking, Irish drinking appears to derive much of its enjoyment from the state of intoxication – many Irish drinkers drink to get drunk. Irish society appears unusually tolerant of drunkenness. In *The Playboy of the Western World*, Pegeen Mike's father provides a telling account of the solemnity and significance of drunkenness when, in extolling the virtues of the funeral wake he has just attended, he remarks, 'You'd never seen the match of it for flows of drink, the way we sunk her bones at noonday in her narrow grave, there were five men, aye and six men stretched out retching speechless on the holy stones.'

This tolerance stretches to our legislation. We permit people to drive cars with as much as 80 milligrams of alcohol per 100 millilitres of blood, whereas the legal limit in Britain and France is 50. In Sweden it is 20 and in Finland and Norway, zero.

ALCOHOLISM, HEAVY AND PROBLEM DRINKING
The term 'alcoholic' has become the single greatest obstacle to a sensible, informed public debate in Ireland about the use and misuse of alcohol. While most people do not have a clear, informed opinion of what constitutes an alcoholic – other than the certainty that they themselves are not one – we appear to

assume that it is only 'alcoholics' who have to worry about their patterns of drinking and their attitudes to alcohol. This is quite erroneous. First, there is the fact that the overwhelming majority of alcohol-related problems in our society are caused by people who are not alcoholic, but who are drinking heavily or inappropriately. Road traffic fatalities are a good example. Two-thirds of people who die in Irish traffic accidents – pedestrians as well as drivers, passengers and motorcyclists – have levels of alcohol in their blood that are well in excess of our generous legal limit. The great majority of these people are not alcoholic. Yet the problems caused in such accidents – death, mutilation, permanent disability, protracted, expensive and avoidable hospitalisation, prolonged legal proceedings and loss of productivity – are alcohol-related and people who produce them are rightly regarded as misusing alcohol.

The term 'alcoholic' is reserved for those individuals who have become physically dependent on alcohol to such an extent that withdrawal of the drug leads to unpleasant physical and psychological experiences – so-called 'withdrawal symptoms'. Why some individuals and not others become physically dependent on alcohol is still not completely understood, but key factors include a genetic and familial predisposition and a persistent exposure to prolonged periods of heavy consumption. In other words, some people are more vulnerable to becoming addicted than others, because of their genetic and psychological make-up, but any of us, if we should drink enough, could become addicted.

'Alcoholism' is a confusing term with off-putting connotations of vagrancy, 'meths' drinking and social disintegration. It has recently been replaced by the term 'alcohol dependence syndrome', which has seven essential elements:

• There is a compulsive need to drink.

• A stereotyped pattern of drinking is established. Whereas the ordinary drinker varies his/her daily pattern, the addicted drinker drinks at regular intervals to avoid or relieve withdrawal symptoms.

13

• Drinking takes primacy over other activities. For the dependent drinker, the day revolves around drinking. Drinking becomes central rather than incidental to the drinker's personal and social life.

• Tolerance to alcohol is altered. The dependent drinker is ordinarily unaffected by blood alcohol levels that would incapacitate a normal drinker. Increasing tolerance is an important sign of increasing dependence. In the later stages of dependence, tolerance suddenly falls.

• There are repeated withdrawal symptoms. These occur some eight to twelve hours after cessation of drinking or after a sharp fall in blood alcohol in people who have been drinking heavily for years. They often appear on waking as a result of the fall in blood alcohol level during sleep.

• Relief drinking. Many dependent drinkers take a drink early in the morning to stave off withdrawal symptoms. In most cultures, including our own, early morning drinking is indicative of alcohol dependence.

• Reinstatement after abstinence is common. A severely dependent drinker who drinks again after a period of abstinence is likely to relapse quickly and return to his/her old addictive pattern.

Problem drinkers are those who cause or experience physical, psychological and/or social harm as a consequence of drinking alcohol. Many problem drinkers, while heavy drinkers, are not psychologically or physically dependent on alcohol. Heavy drinkers are those who drink significantly more in terms of quantity and/or frequency than the average drinker. Binge drinkers are those who drink excessively in short bouts, usually 24-48 hours long, separated by often quite lengthy periods of abstinence. Their overall monthly or weekly alcohol intake may be relatively modest.

SAFE DRINKING

To recognise the drinker who is at risk, it is necessary to have some notion of what constitutes safe drinking. As a result of research, it is now possible to provide a general guide to sensible drinking, summarised as follows.

Guide to Sensible Drinking

- Daily maximum
    - 3 units for men
    - 2 units for women
  To help achieve this:
    - Use a standard measure.
    - Do not drink during the day.
- Have alcohol-free days each week.
- Remember –
    - Health can be damaged without being 'drunk'.
    - Regular heavy intake is more physically damaging than occasional binges.
    - Binges can cause considerable psychological and social problems.
    - Do not drink to 'drown your problems'.
- A unit of alcohol is equivalent to
    - $^1/_2$ pint of beer *or*
    - 1 single measure of spirits *or*
    - 1 glass of wine

WOMEN AND ALCOHOL

Until recently, women were much less at risk of developing alcohol-related problems than men, but there are now signs of a change. In 1988, for example, there were 5147 male admissions to psychiatric hospitals for alcohol-related disorders, compared with 1331 female admissions – nearly five times more men than women. The Irish Psychiatric Hospital Census taken on a specific night – 31 March 1991 — revealed 291 men and 117 women in hospital with a diagnosis of alcohol abuse, a ratio of approximately 2:1.

Clinical opinion is that alcohol problems are increasing in women, which may in turn reflect the changing role and greater personal independence of women, as well as changes in affluence and attitudes. There is, however, evidence that women are in trouble with alcohol for a shorter period before coming for or being brought to treatment than men. So before we conclude that women are having more problems with alcohol than before, it would be necessary to make sure that this was not a consequence of a greater degree of tolerance towards male abuse and intolerance towards female abuse.

Women are advised not to drink alcohol at all during pregnancy, as even small amounts of alcohol can lead to small babies. Larger amounts of alcohol have been linked with foetal abnormalities.

DETECTION OF ALCOHOL-RELATED PROBLEMS

Anyone drinking regularly above sensible drinking guidelines risks developing alcohol-related problems. Alcohol abuse should be suspected in any person manifesting any of the following:

• Absenteeism from work on a regular basis.
• Frequent attendances at the doctor for unexplained indigestion, stomach pain or vomiting.
• Complaints of difficulty sleeping, loss of energy and drive, a marked irritability, a fall-off in sexual interest, headaches, disturbances of memory and concentration, and loss of appetite with or without loss of weight.
• Hospital admissions for accidents of all kinds.
• 'Fits', 'turns' or 'falls'.

A number of questionnaires, such as the CAGE questionnaire (see opposite), have been developed to help identify people with alcohol-related problems. Two or more positive replies to the CAGE questionnaire are said to identify problem drinkers. There are also a number of so-called 'at risk' factors involved, which include:

• Marital difficulties – these may conceal heavy drinking or, more frequently, may be used to justify it.

- Work problems – alcohol abusers have two to three times more days off work than their more sober colleagues.
- An affected relative – 25 per cent of the male relatives of people abusing alcohol have similar problems.
- High risk occupations – these include company directors, salesmen, doctors, journalists, publicans and seamen.

The CAGE questionnaire*

1. Have you ever felt you ought to CUT down on your drinking?
2. Have people ANNOYED you by criticising your drinking?
3. Have you ever felt bad or GUILTY about your drinking?
4. Have you ever had a drink first thing in the morning (an 'EYE-OPENER') to get rid of a hangover?

*From Mayfield D, McLeod G, and Hall P (1974) *American Journal of Psychiatry* 131: 1121-1123. With permission.

Changes in blood and urinary levels of alcohol and in a number of important liver enzymes also help doctors detect people who are abusing alcohol. However, the problem for many friends and relatives is not the detection of alcohol abuse so much as what can be done when alcohol abuse is clearly suspected. Most people in our culture pride themselves on their self-control. We all like to believe that we are using alcohol sensibly. The image of the alcohol abuser is such a negative one that we strongly resist any suggestion that we ourselves might not be drinking sensibly despite evidence to the contrary. Hence denial is a key aspect of the problem. The drinker in trouble almost invariably denies their drinking is harmful, even in the face of mounting problems at home and at work, both physical and mental. A heavy-drinking spouse is inevitably caught up in marital problems which he or she often sees as the cause rather than the consequence of the drinking. In the Irish setting, alcohol problems are much more frequently the cause than the consequence, but it takes many drinkers a considerable period before this can be acknowledged. Other early and worrying signs include financial difficulties as a result of increased spending on alcohol, work difficulties due to impaired concentration, memory impairment, a deterioration in efficiency, and difficulties in getting on with colleagues, particularly if they suspect that drink is a problem.

In general, no favours are done to the person abusing alcohol when family, relatives and friends ignore the fact. The earlier the abuse of alcohol is pointed out to an individual, the better the long-term prognosis. Too often people collude with heavy drinking, hoping it will clear up spontaneously. Confronting someone with their abusive drinking is difficult, particularly since it invariably provokes hostility and denial. In the long term, however, positive confrontation is to be encouraged. It is often helpful to enlist the help of someone who is particularly close to the drinker. In addition, a spouse or family member is advised to seek the help of the family doctor and, if needs be, of a member of Alcoholics Anonymous. AA, the major voluntary movement in this area, has branches and meetings all over Ireland and provides support not merely for alcohol abusers themselves but for the spouses and children of alcohol abusers through its sister movements, Al-Ateen and ACOA (the Adult Children of Alcoholics).

Alcohol abuse in a parent should be suspected in any case where a child appears to be emotionally or physically deprived. One of the saddest consequences of alcoholism in the family is its impact on the confidence and self-esteem of the children. Research has shown that children of alcoholics often manifest severely impaired self-esteem when they in turn become adults. Such children are much more prone to anxiety, depression, and sexual and marital difficulties. In turn, they too may turn to alcohol for the relief of these feelings, thereby completing a particularly vicious and destructive cycle of behaviour.

THE TREATMENT OF ALCOHOL ABUSE

Successful identification of alcohol abuse at an early stage constitutes an important treatment in its own right. It can lead to the provision of factual information concerning safe drinking levels, a recommendation to cut down, and simple support and advice concerning associated problems. Such an approach, which can be delivered by a family doctor or a counsellor, has been found to be as effective as more expensive and specialised forms of psychotherapy in the treatment of drinking which, while heavy, is not addictive.

With addictive drinking, however, more specialised treatment is usually required. Group therapy is one of the most favoured approaches. This involves identification, confession, emotional arousal, the implantation of new ideas and the long-term support of other members of the group. Family and marital therapy involving both alcohol abuser and spouse are also important elements in modern treatment.

Addicted drinkers often experience considerable difficulty when they attempt to reduce or stop their drinking. Withdrawal symptoms are a particular problem and some experience so-called *delirium tremens* (DTs). This may occur between one and five days after cessation of drinking. Sufferers become disorientated, agitated, and have a marked tremor or shake affecting hands and sometimes legs. They experience dramatic and terrifying visual hallucinations, with profuse sweating, rapid pulse and fever. The state requires hospitalisation and medical treatment. Long-term treatment with tranquillising drugs is not favoured in alcohol dependence. But if there is an associated psychiatric condition requiring drug treatment, such as severe depression, it should be treated.

Drugs such as disulfiram (Antabuse) can be used to help the addicted drinker to abstain from alcohol. The drug does not cure dependency but provides a powerful deterrent. It reacts with alcohol to cause very unpleasant side-effects, including flushing, headache, chest tightening and marked apprehension. A daily maintenance dose of such a drug means that an alcohol-dependent drinker must wait until the disulfiram is eliminated from the body before he/she can drink safely. Such drugs, therefore, can provide a 'chemical fence' around the drinker for at least twenty-four hours. They can be helpful in strengthening the motivation of the drinker who seriously desires sobriety but who is given to impulsive changes of mind.

In the case of non-dependent heavy drinkers, the goal of normal drinking within safe limits can be a very reasonable one. However, the alcohol-dependent drinker must be persuaded to abstain from drink totally. Abstention, particularly after many years of drinking, is a difficult goal and, not surprisingly, many fail in the attempt at least initially. Research suggests that between 40 per cent and 50 per cent of alcohol-dependent drinkers are abstinent or drinking very much less up to two years following treatment. Specialised treatment units, psychiatric treatment, group therapy and attendance at AA meetings are all powerful elements in the struggle to keep the alcohol-dependent individual abstinent and healthy.

YOUNG PEOPLE AND ALCOHOL

Irish society, like every western society, has problems with its use of alcohol. Few people recognise its potential for harm until it is too late. Few know the most basic information concerning safe and unsafe amounts and patterns of drinking. If we are to develop a more balanced approach, a number of changes in personal and social behaviour may be required. These might include the following.

• Give children a graded exposure to alcohol within the setting of a strong family unit.

At present, our young people get little coherent guidance concerning alcohol. They are caught between the ideal of abstinence, often with religious connotations, and a social reality in which intoxication is not only tacitly condoned but actively encouraged. More and more young people drink alcohol, and a growing proportion can be found in heavy-drinking statistics and in hospital samples. Accordingly, exhorting young people to abstain while leaving them exposed to peer pressures, advertising blandishments and poor parental guidance and example means that we risk having the worst of both worlds – a heavy-drinking youth culture that is guilty and ambivalent about it.

• Encourage low- and non-alcohol beverages and discourage beverages high in alcohol content.

The main problem with alcoholic drinks is not the volume of the drink that is consumed, but the volume of the alcohol. It is often mistakenly believed, for example, that beer drinking is safe and that it is only spirit drinking that should provoke concern. By virtue of their higher alcohol content, spirits do pose problems, but many heavy drinkers who restrict themselves to beer more than compensate for beer's lower alcohol content by drinking substantial quantities.

• Parents must provide a more consistent example to their children in terms of their own drinking patterns.

Parents too often express their concern about their children's teenage drinking while remaining oblivious to the impact which their own drinking has on these same children. Adults who drink and drive, who themselves become drunk at important family and social occasions and who exhibit indifference to the consequences of over-indulgence in alcohol, are poorly placed to advise their own children and are particularly at risk of encouraging aberrant patterns of drinking in their children.

• Moralising about alcohol abuse might be usefully avoided, but placing a moral taboo on intoxication might help us as a society to develop a more mature and consistent attitude to alcohol.

Drinking *per se* should neither be categorised as a virtue nor as a sin. There has been a tendency in Irish society to see drinking as 'bad' behaviour, thereby encouraging guilt, denial and immature behaviour concerning alcohol. It is not using alcohol but abusing alcohol that should concern us.

———————————————

Professor Anthony Clare MD, FRCPI, FRCPsych, MPhil is the Medical Director of St Patrick's Hospital, Dublin, and Clinical Professor of Psychiatry at Trinity College, Dublin.

ALLERGIES

DR PAUL CARSON

It is often easy to spot someone who suffers from an allergy. The giveaway signs might be red eyes, itchy skin, a streaming nose or a bulge on the hip (caused by a pocketful of soggy tissues)!

There are, however, many people who have hidden allergies which can be much harder to identify and much more difficult to deal with. There are many others who put themselves on odd diets because of a mistaken idea that they are allergic to everyday foods such as wheat and dairy products.

Dr Paul Carson is in general practice. He runs allergy and asthma clinics and has also written a number of books on the subject . . .

Allergies are on the increase. The number of people suffering from allergic asthma and eczema shows a steady upward trend. Between the 1950s and 1980s, there was a fourfold jump in those experiencing summer hay fever. The reasons behind this are not absolutely clear, but some doctors believe that environmental pollution plays an important role.

There is also an increased public awareness of allergy as a major cause of ill health, so a great deal of interest in the subject has arisen. Unfortunately, not all the information available on the topic is necessarily correct, causing confusion and bewilderment to many.

WHAT IS AN ALLERGY?

An allergy is an unusual and exaggerated reaction to a substance that is either inhaled, swallowed, injected, or comes into direct contact with the skin or eyes. Take a simple example. In the middle of June, grass pollen is released into the atmosphere in great quantities. Some unfortunate individuals are exquisitely sensitive to the pollen grains and show allergic reactions. While others are basking in the warm sunshine, these people are so affected that they have to stay indoors to avoid sniffing, sneezing or itching. They are allergy sufferers, and the reactions they show are the exaggerated responses of the body's defence system to the pollen.

Approximately 20 per cent of the population have an inherited potential to develop allergies, although only about half of this group are sufficiently troubled to seek medical help. The allergic state is passed from one generation to the next. If one parent has an allergy, there is twice the chance of their children also developing an allergy. If both parents are allergic, the possibility that their children will be similarly affected is quadrupled.

HOW DO ALLERGIES SHOW UP?

Allergic reactions occur in response to substances that are inhaled, swallowed, injected, or come into direct contact with the skin and eyes.

Inhaled

Hay fever sufferers are allergic to pollen. When the pollen grains are inhaled directly into the nose and lungs, their normally smooth linings swell and produce a mucus-type fluid. This causes blockage in the nose, sneezing and a watery discharge. In the lungs, the same type of swelling and mucus production causes coughing, wheezing and shortness of breath.

Swallowed

Some individuals are extremely sensitive to certain foods such as shellfish. Within minutes of eating it, they start to feel sick and may develop a severe wheeze and a dramatic skin rash. Occasionally they may even collapse.

Injected

Aspirin and related drugs can cause problems for some allergy sufferers. If one of these compounds is injected, a severe and potentially fatal asthmatic attack can occur. Penicillin can also cause a severe allergic reaction, resulting in a rash or swelling of the face and throat.

Direct skin contact

Nickel is a metal that is widely used in jewellery manufacturing. Some people are allergic to it, so if they wear any jewellery containing nickel they will break out in an itchy, red rash where the contact between skin and metal occurs.

These are the four main routes by which substances provoke allergic reactions. Unfortunately, some allergy sufferers can show nearly all of these responses and the quality of their lives can be poor if they do not receive proper help.

WHAT CAUSES ALLERGIES?

The most common allergens (substances causing allergy) are grass and tree pollens, the house dust mite (a microscopic insect found mainly in household dust), animal danders (the hair/scurf/fur/urine shed by animals when it is broken into a dust-type particle), certain metals, wasp and bee venom, drugs and certain foods. There is a popular misconception that foods, especially dairy products, cause most allergy problems, but this is far from the truth.

WHAT ARE THE MAIN ALLERGIC CONDITIONS?

The most common allergic reactions occur in the nose/sinuses and lungs. This is usually in response to dust mites, pollens and/or animal danders. As these enter the nose and are carried into the sinuses, there is swelling of the lining, itching, fluid production and feelings of congestion. Further inhaled into the lungs, the same allergic reaction occurs, causing cough, wheeze and shortness of breath. The link between the nose/sinuses and lungs is important as the lung symptoms (asthma) are often treated while the nose/sinus symptoms are ignored. This can leave allergy sufferers very uncomfortable, going around as if they have a constant head cold. In addition, untreated nasal/sinus allergies can contribute to ongoing asthma. (The subject of asthma is dealt with more fully in the chapter, 'Coughs and Wheezes'.)

Doctors often consider the nose and sinuses as separate from the lungs when dealing with patients. The nose/sinuses are called the upper airways while the lungs are called the lower airways. While it is convenient to keep these areas apart in terms of treatment, they are very much interrelated from an allergy viewpoint.

If you have an allergic nature and are allergic to one or more of the many inhaled allergens (dust mites, pollens, animal danders), there is then a very good chance that you will experience nose and sinus problems. These might be dramatic and obvious, as when someone is suddenly exposed to one of these allergens in high quantities. The hay fever/grass pollen link is a good example again. When pollen production is at its height, hay fever sufferers experience snuffling, sneezing and a runny, itchy nose. Our sinuses are linked directly to the inside lining of the nose and consequently pollen grains can be carried inside them, where a similar allergy occurs. This produces a feeling of congestion around the face. The connection between these symptoms and midsummer is so obvious that there is little doubt about the diagnosis.

However, some allergy sufferers are unaware that the feeling of having a constant head cold is in fact allergy-based. This is usually in response to something to which they are repeatedly exposed, such as dust mites or animal danders. Here the features tend to be of a continuous nasal blockage, a nasal twang to the voice, the constant use of paper tissues and a general nasal irritability. Associated sinus symptoms include a facial pain which is occasionally felt along the upper teeth and behind the eyes. If left unchecked, this constant allergy can lead to nasal polyps.

Nasal polyps are grape-like swellings that develop in the nose and cause great discomfort. Surgery is frequently required to remove them. Because of potential links between the nose/sinuses and the lungs, it is possible that untreated upper airway allergies can contribute to asthma. For this reason, many doctors will include a thorough evaluation of the nose and sinuses as part of an overall assessment of patients with asthma. Allergy testing will confirm whether or not these symptoms are indeed due to an allergy. Sensible decisions can then be made about avoiding exposure.

Allergic reactions affecting the eyes are also common, most obviously during the pollen season for hay fever sufferers. There is intense itching, tearing, even a frightening-looking jelly-like swelling of the whites of the eyes. While this seasonal connection makes the condition easy to diagnose, some people have a more subtle reaction. For them, there is a constant eye irritation, with redness and a general gritty feeling. This can often be tracked down to a repeated exposure to dust mites or animal danders.

Allergies can also affect the skin, causing redness, blistering, itch and scaling. The two most common skin allergies are eczema (also called dermatitis) and urticaria (hives).

Eczema is either of the contact variety (as with nickel sensitivity) or the atopic form. 'Atopic' means 'allergic', and in

27

THE CHECK UP GUIDE TO GOOD HEALTH

long-standing atopic eczema, doctors will often look for underlying allergic causes. This may involve special dietary restrictions and/or methods of reducing exposure to inhaled allergens such as dust mites or animal danders.

Urticaria (hives) can be of the direct contact variety or may possibly be diet-related. Direct contact means that handling something to which you are allergic will produce an itchy skin weal. The connection is so obvious that no tests are needed to identify the problem allergen. A simple example occurs when someone is allergic to cats; if a cat licks the hand, an itchy weal develops. In long-standing non-contact urticaria, a diet avoiding what are known as salicyclates may be suggested as part of treatment. This means avoiding aspirin and aspirin-related medicines, non-steroidal anti-inflammatory drugs (eg Ponstan and Brufen) and many food additives and colourings (eg E102, E104 etc). Your doctor will advise you.

The next most common allergies involve reactions to medicines. These can produce a variety of symptoms such as skin rashes and breathing difficulties. There is usually a straightforward cause-and-effect relationship in which the allergic reaction (of whatever nature) occurs only when the offending medicine is taken and clears as soon as the medicine is stopped. Allergy tests are not used in these situations. The only approach is for sufferers to avoid the medicine that causes the problem. In addition, they should wear a Medic-Alert bracelet (available from the pharmacy) with details of what medicines they are allergic to so that these are never given by mistake.

Wasps and bees cause problems for a small minority of patients who can have allergic reactions to their stings. These reactions vary from local swelling and itch to a generalised, life-threatening reaction. Such patients need to be allergy tested and a treatment programme planned to avert such severe reactions.

WHEN DO ALLERGIES START?

Allergies can start at any age, but most develop in childhood before the age of five. The nature of the allergy can change over time. For instance, a young child may begin with a skin reaction such as eczema, then go on to develop asthma. At the age of ten or eleven, the allergy may manifest itself as hay fever. By the time the person reaches their twenties or thirties, they may have developed nasal polyps.

Some people have more than one type of allergic reaction. Asthma and eczema often go together, as do asthma and hay fever, while some people unfortunately have multiple reactions and suffer from asthma, eczema and nasal polyps.

WHAT ABOUT FOOD ALLERGIES?

Most people with allergies believe that their symptoms are due to something they eat or drink. But for the majority, inhaled allergens such as dust mites, pollens and animal danders are by far the most important causes of allergy. Indeed people's perception and misinterpretation of foods/drinks as being allergy-provoking often lead them to strange diets which rarely bring about any improvement.

Food and drink can affect individuals in a variety of ways, although not all of them result in allergic reactions. If you do have a true food allergy, you will be advised to avoid that particular food totally, so it is as well to be certain before restricting your diet.

Let's look at some examples in which people mistakenly feel they are allergic to a particular food/drink. If you drink too much coffee, you might get palpitations. This is not an allergy to coffee but a response to too much caffeine in the coffee stimulating the heart rate. You can comfortably drink coffee in lesser quantities. If you drink too much gin you will get drunk and end up with a hangover. This is not an allergy to gin, but the result of an accumulation of too much alcohol and the effect it has on the body. You can drink gin in small quantities and not get drunk. However, if you are truly allergic to certain foods/drinks, even small quantities will produce unpleasant allergic reactions. Avoidance is the only sensible option.

True food allergy usually occurs in an immediate or delayed

fashion. 'Immediate' implies that the adverse reaction happens quickly, usually within a short time of the food entering the stomach. Indeed some food allergy reactions occur as soon as the food crosses the lips, causing swelling, intense itching and rashes to appear on the lips and mouth. This is very often seen in children with, for example, an egg allergy; the egg rarely gets further than their mouth before the reaction begins. In this situation, the response is so immediate and dramatic that the child and his/her parents learn not to try that food again.

Other forms of immediate reactions can be very dramatic, even life-threatening, if the offending food enters the stomach. Severe and violent vomiting can occur, accompanied by dramatic skin rashes and intense wheezing. The sufferer may experience a sudden drop in blood pressure, causing him/her to collapse. This type of reaction is seen mainly with cow's milk (in infants), nuts, eggs, fish and shellfish; other foods (cereal grains, chocolate and citrus fruits) have also been incriminated. In these forms of true food allergy, avoidance is the only form of treatment. Typically, these reactions are fairly severe and occur at intervals, but only when the suspect food is eaten. They are often recognised by the patients themselves. People who have dramatic reactions to Brazil nuts or peanuts, for example, need to be extremely careful to avoid them. Peanuts are often incorporated into manufactured or restaurant foods where they are least anticipated. For this reason, some patients who have had one very bad reaction will be advised to carry a special resuscitation injection with them which they have to administer in an emergency.

While some forms of allergies such as urticaria may disappear spontaneously, these very dramatic food allergies may persist for a long time and may never go away.

Delayed reactions to foods/drinks are more difficult to identify because the delay between consuming the food and the resultant symptoms can vary from hours to days. When a reaction occurs, your doctor has to try and unravel this time warp to determine whether it is due to something consumed today, yesterday or even the day before. Conditions where delayed responses of an allergic nature occur include allergic (atopic) eczema, asthma, migraine, urticaria (hives), angio-oedema (a first cousin to urticaria but of a more dramatic type with swelling of the lips and eyes), epilepsy (but rarely), a few well-defined intestinal conditions, and hyperactive behaviour in children.

Hyperactivity is a rather controversial problem in which children show bizarre and often uncontrollable behaviour patterns. The result is often hell on earth for their parents who will clutch at any straws in the search for help. Over the years, there have been exaggerated claims for the role of food allergy in hyperactive children and rather restrictive diets have been recommended. The truth is that only a small minority of hyperactive children show any lasting improvement after they have been put on a specific diet. Those who don't respond to diet changes may need a programme of behaviour therapy under the guidance of a child psychologist or trained counsellor.

HOW DO WE FIND OUT WHAT WE ARE ALLERGIC TO?

The obvious answer is to do an allergy test. There are two commonly used and acceptable allergy tests: blood testing, and a procedure called skin prick testing.

In blood testing, a sample of blood is taken from the patient and sent to a laboratory for analysis. One type of test checks the general allergy level (called total IgE), while another (called a RAST test) looks for specific substances to which one might be allergic. As these tests are expensive and time-consuming, many doctors are reluctant to order them unless absolutely necessary.

The second test, the skin prick test, is simpler and much less expensive to perform. In addition, the results can be obtained within thirty minutes while the patient waits.

In the skin prick test, drops of each substance your doctor wishes to check are placed on the forearm. The skin is then gently pricked underneath the drop so that the extract comes into direct contact with the cells exposed in the pricked skin. If you are allergic to any of the tested extracts, an intensely itchy weal

31

forms on the skin. The size and shape of this weal reflects the strength of the allergy. By the end of the test, there is an accurate picture of a person's allergic state and the substances to which they are allergic. Skin prick testing is regarded as accurate and correctly reflects an allergic condition. In some delayed forms of food allergy, however, neither the skin prick nor blood sample test will pick up the offending food. A special restrictive diet is then used, with suspect foods introduced gradually and reactions noted.

In a contact skin allergy, a patch test is used to determine what is causing the problem. This involves placing various test materials directly onto the skin and holding them in place with elastoplast. Any reaction is read after forty-eight hours and takes the form of a red, itchy area of skin.

If you are allergic, or if you suspect that you have an allergy, you should go to a reputable centre for investigation and treatment. Unfortunately, some alternative health practitioners perform allergy tests that have been consistently shown to be bogus and useless. Occasionally, health food shops offer allergy-testing services. Beware of these as well. The following are the most common alternative allergy tests used in this country: hair analysis, Vega testing, applied kinesiology, pulse increase test and dowsing. All of them are totally useless and will give no help in allergy diagnosis and treatment.

HOW DO DOCTORS HELP
ALLERGY SUFFERERS?

Identification

Is your health problem due to an allergy? If so, what are you allergic to? You must first check with a doctor and have an allergy test.

Avoidance

Depending on the result of your allergy test, a special diet may be suggested, perhaps along with the recommendation that you avoid those environments in which you will find the substances to which you are allergic. Special actions to reduce dust mite exposure are occasionally recommended. These include: removing carpets, feather pillows and woollen blankets from bedrooms; vacuuming carpets, curtains and bedding regularly; and using Banamite spray (available from pharmacies) to kill dust mites. It can take up to three months for these measures to work and to show definite benefits.

Treatment

Anti-allergy medicines may be prescribed to relieve symptoms, especially if you suffer from allergic asthma, eczema or allergies affecting the nose and sinuses. One group of anti-allergy medicines now freely available without prescription are called antihistamines. In the past, these drugs had a bad reputation as they caused marked drowsiness. It was a toss-up as to which was worse, the condition or the treatment! Now, however, there are excellent preparations which are free from these side-effects (eg Triludan or Clarityn) and which are very useful in conditions such as hay fever and urticaria. Although they are of little use in asthma, they give some help in year-round allergic rhinitis and may help a little in eczema. If you buy antihistamines from the pharmacy without a doctor's advice, you should try them for no more than a week. If there is no real improvement in that time, have your doctor review the situation in case the problem is not allergy-related at all.

Desensitisation

This implies a special form of injection therapy. A course of injections containing exactly what you are allergic to is given, but in very small, dilute doses. The idea is to stimulate your own natural immunity so that you stop reacting in an allergic manner when exposed again to whatever is in the treatment programme. This regime is useful in nasal allergy (allergic rhinitis), mild allergic asthma and allergy to stinging insects. Because of very strict rules governing who can administer this treatment and where, it may be difficult to obtain outside of a hospital setting.

For the majority of allergy sufferers, the programme of identification, avoidance and appropriate treatment with anti-allergy medicines is all that is needed. So put away those tissues, stop sniffling and scratching! Get along to your family doctor for help.

Dr Paul Carson BA, MB, BCh, BAO, DFPA is a GP in Dublin where he runs an asthma and allergy clinic for children. He is the author of a series of four books dealing with allergy problems in children and is a member of the British Society for Allergy and Clinical Immunology.

ARTHRITIS AND RHEUMATISM

DR OLIVER FITZGERALD

Approximately a quarter of all adults suffer from aches and pains in their muscles and joints every year. Arthritis is one of the most common conditions known to man and it is the biggest single cause of disability. Over 100,000 people in Ireland are disabled because of arthritis. So it is not surprising that it has been described as 'Ireland's biggest pain'.

Consultant rheumatologist Dr Oliver FitzGerald describes the various forms of arthritis, the difference between arthritis and rheumatism, and how modern treatment can relieve pain and prevent disability . . .

WHAT IS ARTHRITIS?

Many patients who consult their doctors about aches and pains and who are concerned about the possibility of arthritis do not, in fact, have arthritis. The word 'arthritis' means inflammation in the joints. The features of inflammation are pain, swelling, heat, redness and loss of joint function. Joint pain on its own may not indicate arthritis. The pain may be coming from the tissues and structures around the joints (tendons and ligaments), rather than from the joints themselves. The presence of joint swelling is of particular importance when making a diagnosis of arthritis.

A joint is where two opposing bones move, one on top of the other. The joint surface is lined by a white, gristly substance known as cartilage, which provides a smooth surface for the opposing bone to move on. The joint is encased in a strong ligament-type structure called the joint capsule. The inner aspect of the capsule is lined by a structure called the synovial membrane which is normally a very thin clingfilm-like structure which helps to lubricate the joint. Inside the joint cavity, a small amount of fluid known as synovial fluid is normally present.

TYPES OF ARTHRITIS

Arthritis can broadly be broken into four groups: osteoarthritis, rheumatoid arthritis, ankylosing spondylitis and others. It is important to remember that arthritis is not just a feature of increasing age, as the condition can begin at any age, even during childhood. It is not commonly appreciated that there are many children in Ireland who are suffering from juvenile chronic arthritis.

Osteoarthritis

Osteoarthritis is primarily a disease of the cartilage which initially develops fissures and cracks and which gradually becomes worn and irregular. The exact cause of osteoarthritis is not known. While osteoarthritis may occur in the younger population following such conditions as congenital deformities of the hip or following trauma (injury), it is generally a condition of the older population, beginning particularly in the fifth and sixth decades. Women are more commonly affected than men. The joints involved include those at the tips of the fingers, the base of the thumb, the neck and lower spine, the large weight-bearing joints of the hips and knees, and the base of the big toe. Patients generally complain of gradually increasing discomfort, stiffness and a limitation of movement. Joint swelling may be a feature and the swelling is often hard and bony.

Osteoarthritis is very common and in most patients it progresses slowly, if at all. While joints may have symptoms from time to time, most patients maintain full function and their joints may only require intermittent attention. The occasional patient with osteoarthritis has more severe symptoms, and disability may occur, particularly with severe involvement of the hips or knees. In the early stages, treatment is aimed at relieving symptoms with pain-killers or intermittent anti-inflammatory medication and physiotherapy to maintain range of movement. If the disease is more severe, joint replacement surgery may be indicated. Hip and knee surgery in particular are now so successful that the patient may have a completely new lease of life. Patients who are almost wheelchair-bound can become mobile, pain-free and independent again.

Rheumatoid arthritis

In contrast to osteoarthritis, rheumatoid arthritis affects patients predominantly in their forties and fifties, although it can commence at any age. Again, females are more commonly affected than males, and with a prevalence rate of approximately 1 per cent of the population, it is reasonable to estimate that there are 30,000 cases of rheumatoid arthritis in Ireland alone. Commonly, patients present with the gradual onset of pain, swelling and limitation of movement affecting the small joints of the hands and feet, with the knees, wrists and ankles also frequently involved. For reasons not fully understood, the same joints on both sides of the body are often affected, for example the same fingers, which is sometimes a useful feature for diagnosis. Patients may also complain of non-specific symptoms

37

such as fatigue, weight loss or malaise (a general feeling of being unwell).

The course of rheumatoid arthritis is variable, and the disease is characterised by fluctuating symptoms and signs which make it difficult to assess the effects of any particular treatment. Up to 30 per cent of patients may undergo a spontaneous and complete improvement in their symptoms, and these remissions may be quite prolonged. The course in a further 30 per cent of patients is one of recurrent flare-ups and remissions, with the patient generally returning to full function in between attacks. Finally, there is a group of patients in whom the disease tends to pursue a slow, insidious course with increasing joint damage and disability over time. These patients need to be identified early and treated to control joint inflammation and to prevent any joint damage.

In rheumatoid arthritis, the primary abnormality is in the thin synovial membrane which becomes markedly inflamed and which gradually invades and causes damage to the underlying joint cartilage. In the early stages of disease, the cartilage is quite normal. If the synovial membrane inflammation can be controlled at this stage, progression to joint deformity can be prevented.

Ankylosing spondylitis
Unlike other forms of arthritis, ankylosing spondylitis is predominantly a disease of males which most commonly begins in one's twenties or thirties. Patients generally complain of the gradual onset of low back pain and stiffness. These are usually worse after rest and are often relieved by exercise. Mainly a disease of the spine, it particularly affects the joints at the base of the spine, the sacro-iliac joints. Other joints may be involved in about 30 per cent of patients, including the large weight-bearing joints of the hips and knees. Because of the pain and inflammation in the spine, the tendency is towards loss of movement in the spine over time. Without treatment, spinal movements can become quite restricted, leading to an abnormal stooped posture in more advanced cases.

OTHER FORMS OF ARTHRITIS

Other forms of arthritis that deserve mention include gout, connective tissue disease and psoriatic arthritis.

Gout

Gout has traditionally been associated with too much high living; the picture of the obese man propping his big red toe up on a stool often springs to mind. However, what is not appreciated is that gout can be an extremely painful condition. While alcohol and rich food can contribute to the problem, a genetic predisposition to gout is of more importance. Gout is caused by excessive amounts of uric acid, a normal breakdown product of protein. Inside the joints, the uric acid tends to crystalise. This can result in the joints becoming very inflamed. If left untreated, gout can be debilitating, as well as leading to progressive joint deformity. With proper management, it should be possible to prevent both further attacks and joint deformity.

Connective tissue disorders

Connective tissue disorders can also affect the joints. Perhaps the best known of these is a condition called systematic lupus erythematosis (SLE). This is an uncommon disorder in which the joints are frequently inflamed and where there may be involvement of many other organs, particularly the skin. The arthritis in SLE is often mild. Only in occasional patients does it lead to underlying joint damage and subsequent deformity.

Psoriatic arthritis

Psoriatic arthritis sufferers show evidence of joint inflammation in association with the skin rash, psoriasis. This typically produces scaling on the scalp, over the elbows or on the knees. Up to 10 per cent of patients with psoriasis have an associated arthritis. This can vary from involving only a few joints to a condition that involves most of the joints and which is similar to rheumatoid arthritis. In some patients with psoriatic arthritis, the back may be mainly afflicted and the condition may appear similar to ankylosing spondylitis.

RHEUMATISM

About 30 per cent of patients who complain of multiple aches and pains do not have arthritis at all. Instead, their aches and pains relate to the tissues around the joints, such as the ligaments and tendons. These people are thought to suffer from a condition called soft tissue rheumatism, or fibromyalgia. Fibromyalgia sufferers are commonly females in their twenties or thirties. They complain of diffuse aches and pains with no evidence of joint inflammation. Examination reveals multiple areas of soft tissue tenderness. There is commonly an associated fatigue accompanied by sleep disturbance. While stress may play a role in some patients, the underlying sleep disturbance may be a more important factor. Correcting the sleep disturbance certainly seems to help ease the symptoms and improve functioning.

Rheumatism is a term that could also be used to describe localised pain and tenderness such as tennis elbow or tendonitis. These local problems are generally brought on by injury or repetitive strain. Symptoms are usually short-lived and respond to physiotherapy or occasionally to cortisone injections. It is important to find out what factors may be triggering the problem, and where possible, to take corrective measures. For example, tennis elbow is due to an excessive amount of gripping under force. Increasing the size of the instrument gripped may help improve matters.

RISK FACTORS

It is commonly believed that the incidence of arthritis in Ireland is higher than elsewhere, and that the weather and diet may be contributing factors. With regard to the weather, the incidence of arthritis appears to be the same here as it is in countries with warmer climates. The cold and the damp may play a role in increasing a patient's symptoms, but they certainly are not the underlying causes of the problem. With regard to diet, patients with arthritis will know that almost everybody they meet will have a pet cure for arthritis. These cures range from avoiding dairy products and citrus fruit to taking cod liver oil and green mussels from New Zealand. If only it were so simple! Unfortunately, there is little scientific evidence to back up these claims. The only useful advice on diet and arthritis is to keep your weight under control and to stick to a nutritious, balanced diet.

Genetic factors are undoubtedly important in determining the likelihood or otherwise of developing arthritis. In ankylosing spondylitis, for example, there is a strong association with a genetic factor found on cells called the HLA B27 antigen. Half of the children with a HLA B27 positive parent will inherit the gene. However, it has been estimated that less than 25 per cent of these will actually develop the disease. It has been suggested, therefore, that there is an environmental factor, possibly a micro-organism, that is responsible for triggering the disease in patients with the appropriate genetic make-up.

Genetic factors also play a role in rheumatoid arthritis, as well as in osteoarthritis where the relationship is not as clear cut but where there is certainly a higher incidence of these forms of arthritis in the relatives of sufferers. Other risk factors include injury and obesity, both of which increase the risk of developing osteoarthritis.

PREVENTION

Prevention of arthritis is mostly about common sense. Avoiding injury and excess weight gain are of obvious importance. It is also essential to pay attention to good posture, both at home and in the workplace, and to use good lifting techniques in order to prevent excess strain on the lower back. This is especially important for people whose occupations involve a lot of heavy lifting.

EXERCISE

In general, common sense should prevail. If exercise is causing pain, there is something wrong and you should seek help. If a joint is swollen and inflamed, rest will help settle it down. But once that has happened, you should exercise to build up muscle mass again.

MANAGEMENT OF ARTHRITIS

It is important to seek medical assistance early in the course of a developing arthritis. Practical steps and medical intervention early on may have important long-term consequences, whereas delay in diagnosis and treatment can make it difficult to achieve much lasting benefit. If patients' symptoms are not responding to simple measures, the GP will often seek a specialist opinion from a consultant rheumatologist. Apart from suggesting changes in medication, the rheumatologist will often co-ordinate a team approach, which usually includes a physiotherapist, an occupational therapist and nursing staff. Some arthritis patients run into employment difficulties and may need the help of a medical social worker or a vocational assessment officer. Psychologists may be able to give useful support to those who have problems in coping with their arthritis. Other medical consultants may also be called in, particularly orthopaedic surgeons when joint replacement is required. Education is also important in helping to allay patients' fears and in helping them to cope with what is often a chronic disease.

FUTURE PROSPECTS FOR TREATMENT

While the current treatments available can do much to relieve patients' symptoms and prevent disease progression, there are now prospects for newer treatments which may be both more specific and more effective. Recent and ongoing research, particularly with rheumatoid arthritis, has helped to identify what is happening to the cells inside an inflamed joint in order to produce new drugs which may arrest the inflammatory response. With preliminary studies of these new treatments already in progress, it is hoped that they may become more generally available in the not-too-distant future.

Useful address

The Arthritis Foundation of Ireland, 1 Clanwilliam Square, Grand Canal Quay, Dublin 2. Tel. (01) 6618188.

The Arthritis Foundation has produced a number of leaflets on different aspects of arthritis. They also stock a range of aids to help those living with arthritis.

Dr Oliver FitzGerald MD, FRCPI, MRCP is a Consultant Rheumatologist at St Vincent's Hospital, Dublin.

BACK PAIN

MR FRANK DOWLING/ MARIE ELAINE GRANT

If you are chatting with any group of people and someone mentions that they have a back problem, the chances are that the conversation will immediately turn to the subject of the bad back. At one time or another, most people will experience back trouble. For many, low back pain is something that they know will return again and again. It may start after a bout of gardening, a long journey, or for no particular reason.

According to orthopaedic surgeon Mr Frank Dowling and chartered physiotherapist Marie Elaine Grant, there is much you can do to keep your spine healthy and avoid injury. They explain the different options for treating low back pain when trouble starts.

LOW BACK PAIN

The most frequently reported and repeated statistic regarding low back pain is that at some point in their lives, some 60-80 per cent of the population will experience low back pain. A significant proportion – 30-70 per cent of those who experience back pain once – will have recurrent problems. Of those who develop a chronic condition and who are off work for longer than six months because of it, only half will ever return to work.

Given the magnitude of this problem, it is important to find ways to prevent it. To do this, the causes must be identified. The structures that work together to form the spine must also be understood.

The spine is made up of twenty-four bones (vertebrae) which are aligned in three flexible curves. Each bone has a solid part in front and a bony arch at the back. The hole in the middle is the canal through which the spinal cord runs from the brain. Between each vertebra is a disc which acts both as a mobile spacer and a shock absorber to cushion the vertebrae during movements such as running or jumping. The outside of the disc is made up of a hard ring of ligament, while the centre is soft and jelly-like. The vertebral arches are joined together above and below by small facet joints. These facet joints are at the back of the spine and on each side of each vertebra.

Nerves leave the spinal cord through small openings between each vertebra. When pressure is placed on a nerve root, as with inflammation or disc protrusion, pain is felt in the nerve pathway supplied by that nerve – such as radiating pain down the leg when there is pressure on the sciatic nerve. This is often referred to as sciatica.

The vertebrae are held together by strong ligaments which run along the front and the back of the spine. There are also ligaments which hold the facet joints together. The abdominal and trunk muscles are also important for allowing movement, holding the spine upright and supporting the spine in a good postural position.

All of these structures are necessary for maintaining a healthy spine. Damage to one part can lead to secondary problems with another part, giving rise to persistent back pain.

CAUSES OF LOW BACK PAIN

In some cases, it is difficult to diagnose exactly why back pain has occurred (non-specific low back pain). Some low back pain is completely unavoidable, such as that caused by congenital abnormalities, spinal tumours, rheumatoid arthritis or other inflammatory diseases. However, the vast majority of back problems arise from mechanical reasons. Many of these mechanical problems can be avoided if you are aware of the risk factors and learn to take care of your back.

Wear and tear or degeneration

Years of poor back management can cause unnecessary wear and tear to the spine, leading to chronic low back pain. With repeated forces placed on the spine, the disc is eventually weakened, leading to a tear in the outer layer. In time, the disc matter protrudes, putting pressure on the nerve root, causing low back pain and often radiating pain into the leg. The disc then begins to flatten, causing the intervertebral disc space to narrow. The bony surfaces of the vertebrae start to grind together as the spine moves, and this causes further wear and tear of the joints. The joint surface becomes roughened, giving rise to tiny bony spurs of the vertebrae. These may then cause further irritation and damage to the spinal nerves.

Disc problems

A slipped disc, or a prolapsed disc as it is more properly called, can arise from wear and tear. The central part of the disc containing the jelly-like substance becomes dried up like crab meat. When the disc is dry, the outer hard rim cracks more easily. The dried gel then oozes out through the crack. As it pushes out of the disc, it causes low back pain. Then, as it presses on a nerve root, it can lead to radiating pain into the leg (sciatica).

A prolapsed disc may also be caused by a sudden tear of the disc, which usually happens when bending, lifting or when bending and twisting at the same time. This can often happen suddenly, in a trivial way, simply by carrying out an awkward movement.

Strains and sprains

Strained ligaments of the spine can occur in one of two ways. The spine may suddenly be twisted or overstretched, as when playing sport. This will result in immediate pain and discomfort. Strain can also occur from overstretching the ligaments due to sustained periods of bad posture. Sitting or standing in a poor postural position for a long time can lead to aching pain in the low back.

Arthritis of posterior facet joints

Degeneration and wear and tear at the intervertebral disc space lead to loss of height at the disc space. This causes telescoping of the posterior facet joint, which becomes malaligned and causes more wear and tear. This leads to joint changes or arthritis of the facet joints. The most common cause of constant low-grade ache in the back, buttocks or hips is due to arthritis of the posterior facet joints.

DIAGNOSING YOUR BACK PROBLEM

The first step towards diagnosing a back problem is through examination by your doctor. Back pain may be a symptom of some other disorder or disease process, including kidney disorders or gynaecological problems. So it is important to ensure that your back pain actually is the result of a low back problem. Physical examination by a doctor can give some indication as to the cause. However, exact causes are difficult to diagnose due to the complexity of the spine. Very often, the following clinical signs can help towards diagnosis.

• Low back pain that is increased by bending or sit-ups is likely to be from a disc.

• Low back pain that is increased by stretching is most likely to be due to arthritis of the posterior facet joints.

• Leg pain that is increased by raising the leg straight is most likely to be due to a slipped disc.

Very often, your doctor will request X-rays as a first line of investigation. X-rays, however, are limited in the information they give about the spine, as they will only show up bony abnormalities. There are various other forms of radiological examinations which will examine specific aspects of the spine in close detail, including discogram, facet arthrograms and CAT (computed tomography) scanning. The most recent development, known as MRI (magnetic resonance imaging) creates an image of a vertical slice through the spine which greatly assists in diagnosing disc degeneration, bulges of the disc and other spinal disorders.

PREVENTING LOW BACK PAIN

It is important to remember that most back problems do not result from a single injury. There are many factors related to our lifestyles and the poor management of our backs that ultimately lead to low back pain. In order to prevent back problems, it is important to maintain a healthy spine.

One of the most effective ways of doing this is to maintain the natural curve of the back in a balanced position. In the lumbar region, there is a small inward curve in the back just above the pelvis. This is known as the lumbar lordosis. To ensure that unnecessary stress is not placed on the lower part of the spine, it is important to maintain the lumbar lordosis in a balanced position. Due to the increased compressive forces of poor posture, damage may be caused to the ligaments and joints of the spine over time.

Standing
Maintenance of a balanced lumbar lordosis is essential. There is a wide variation of normal posture. When standing, your

abdominal muscles pull up in front and the buttock muscles pull down at the back. A spine that has good mobility and strong surrounding muscles adopts a normal posture naturally.

Sitting

Most people who sit for prolonged periods will eventually adopt a poor posture. When you maintain a slouched sitting position, your upper body presses on your lower back, causing overstretching of the ligaments. In time, this may cause the disc joints to become sore.

Travelling a long distance can aggravate a back problem. When driving, stop every hour and walk a little – even walking around the car will help. On a plane, get up every hour or so and walk up and down the aisles. In this way you won't feel so stiff at the end of your journey.

People with sedentary office jobs can easily develop problems as they often sit with a rounded back for hours. You may initially experience very mild low backache after hours of sitting, or you may only experience pain when rising from prolonged sitting. This is caused by overstretching of the soft tissues.

Maintain your spine in its balanced, neutral position by using a chair that supports the three natural curves of your back, particularly your lower back. If the chair does not offer adequate support, you can add support by using a lumbar roll or some other type of back support.

How to choose a good chair

• A seat should always feel comfortable to sit in.

• A chair should give firm (not rigid) back support, including lumbar support, so that a balanced lordosis is maintained while sitting.

• Your seat should be the correct height. While sitting, your feet should rest flat on the floor and your thighs should remain horizontal without pressing into the seat. If the seat is too high to allow your feet to rest flat on the floor, put them on a foot rest, a box or some books.

• The depth of the seat should be less than the distance from the back of the buttocks to behind the knee. If the seat depth is too long or too shallow, it will lead to discomfort and poor posture.

• Most seats are perfectly horizontal, although a slight backward slope may sometimes be useful to allow full use of the back rest, for example a car seat.

• Your desk shouldn't be too high or too low. To judge the correct height, sit straight at your desk, with your arms hanging down by your side. If the desk is level with your elbows, then it is a suitable height for you.

• Arm rests should allow your chair to be pulled in under the desk.

Standing after sitting

After a period of sitting, it is important not to put any strain on the lower back when you stand up. This is particularly relevant if you are suffering from low back ache. Keeping your back straight, move out to the edge of the chair, then push off the chair with your hands while straightening your knees at the same time.

Lying in bed

When sleeping, ensure that your mattress gives adequate support. A mattress should be firm enough to prevent you from sinking into it, yet soft enough to conform to the normal curves of the body. Above all, it should feel comfortable. If your mattress is not giving sufficient support, try placing a board under it. If you suffer from low back pain, sleep in positions that offer your back relief from symptoms and that give good support:

• Lie on your back with one small pillow under your knees and one small pillow under your head and neck.

• Lie on your side. Keep your lower leg nearly straight and bend your top leg. Place a pillow between your legs for greater support.

Overnight, the average spine stretches by up to two centimetres, so the back is most vulnerable in the morning. Be careful when getting out of bed, especially if you are prone to back problems. Instead of jumping up and flinging yourself out of bed, ease yourself out gently by first getting into a sitting position.

BODY MECHANICS FOR LIFTING

When lifting, you can prevent injuries by ensuring that you use safe body mechanics throughout the lift. Keep your back straight and make sure that your lower limbs take the load by bending your knees and hips to squat.

• Plan your lift. Evaluate the weight of the object before trying to lift it. Ensure that there are no obstacles in your way.

• Get as close to the object as possible and keep it close to you while doing the lift.

• Tighten your abdominal muscles and lift the object, keeping your back straight and straightening your knees to lift the load.

• Use your legs to lift the load – always squat down to the object.

• Tighten your stomach muscles while lifting. This helps to maintain the spine in a balanced position.

• Test the weight of the load before attempting to lift. Ask for help when necessary.

• Don't twist your back while lifting. If you need to turn, use your feet to turn. Avoid unnecessary stretching.

• Do not do quick, jerking movements while lifting. Smooth, controlled movements are essential.

• When lowering the object after lifting, again bend your knees and hips. Do not bend your back. Keep your stomach muscles pulled in.

• Always use mechanical help where possible – wheelbarrows, trolleys etc.

The same principles apply for pushing and pulling. Use your legs to take the load. Remember to keep your back straight and to tighten your stomach muscles (do not hold your breath).

OTHER FACTORS THAT CONTRIBUTE
TO BACK PAIN

Poor flexibility, poor muscle strength, reduced fitness and stress are all factors that can increase the possibility of back strain.

Flexibility is the ability of your muscles and ligaments to stretch as you work your joints through a range of movements. If these structures tighten, it makes it more difficult for the joints to adapt to different positions. If you keep your joints flexible, especially in your hips, knees and ankles, your body can adapt to sitting, standing and lifting without putting unwanted strain on your back.

The muscles surrounding the spine keep your back supported and balanced. Weakness in the muscles of the trunk or lower limbs can result in putting unwanted strain on your back. Developing strength in these muscles is important for maintaining a healthy back, especially for people who do a great deal of lifting.

Excess weight puts extra strain on the joints and soft tissues of the back. Being overweight, with sagging stomach muscles, pulls the spine into an unbalanced posture and increases the likelihood of injury.

Poor levels of physical fitness can contribute to general deconditioning and overweight, increasing the risk factors for low back pain. Regular daily exercise such as walking or swimming helps to keep the muscles that support your spine in good condition. Stressful living and work habits can also give rise to low back pain, especially when there is generalised increased muscle tension.

WHAT CAN BE DONE WHEN
PAIN STRIKES?

Back disorders arise for many different reasons. Therefore, the most suitable form of treatment varies from patient to patient. Treatment should always be based on a reasonable diagnosis. Once back pain strikes, ensure that your problem is expertly treated and managed straight away. Neglected back pain can lead to chronic pain.

CONSERVATIVE TREATMENT

Bed rest

Bed rest can be successful for the patient with very acute low back pain. A period of bed rest should only last for a few days – any longer can lead to stiffening in the small joints of the back which will prolong the pain. When taking bed rest for acute low back pain, try to adopt one of the postures described above. After a few days' bed rest, try to return to normal activities slowly, observing all the points of good posture.

Application of heat and cold

A hot bath can relax the muscles and give considerable relief – and help muscle spasm. Localised heat can also be helpful. However, it is not recommended that you use very intense heat. Localised heat should not be applied for more than fifteen minutes at a time. Any longer would cause irritation rather than relief.

Applying cold, for example using crushed ice in a bag or a bag of frozen food, can also help. Cold therapy should be applied for ten minutes at a time. Do not apply for any more than twelve minutes at a time, as any longer may cause ice burns.

Massage

Massage seems more beneficial for people suffering from acutely strained backs than for those with long-standing chronic back problems. Massage applied rhythmically and skilfully can do much to relieve muscle spasm. As far as possible, massage should not cause increased pain, even when massaging tight painful tissue.

Medication

Analgesics (pain-killers) can be used for relief of pain. These can be helpful especially when acute or severe pain strikes. These drugs simply give pain relief but do not remove the causes of back pain.

Anti-inflammatory drugs may be prescribed by your doctor. They act locally on the inflamed (swollen) joints and tissues in the spine. When inflammation is relieved, there is an increased rate of healing and a resulting decrease in pain. Anti-inflammatory gels can be useful for ligament or muscle damage in the back. They are also beneficial in the treatment of acute strains and sprains. They should be used as directed by your doctor or chartered physiotherapist. Gels have an advantage over anti-inflammatory tablets as they do not cause stomach irritation.

Muscle relaxants may also be prescribed by your doctor. They are usually effective in relieving the local back muscle spasm or cramp.

Electrotherapy

Electrotherapy treatments applied by a chartered physiotherapist can be effective in reducing back pain, reducing inflammation, relieving muscle spasm and promoting healing. There are many different forms of electrotherapy available, including shortwave diathermy, ultrasound, interferential, laser, TENS (transcutaneous electrical nerve stimulation), low frequency electrical currents and various forms of heat treatment. The most appropriate treatment for your condition will be decided by your physiotherapist.

Traction

In traction, a stretching force is applied to the spine in order to cause a slight pull on the vertebrae and a prolonged stretching on contracted muscles to relieve muscle spasm. Prolonged periods of traction, along with bed rest, have not been used very widely in recent times as it is thought that a short period of bed rest without traction is just as effective. Intermittent traction applied by a physiotherapist is now the more common form. The most appropriate position, load and frequency of traction will depend on your particular condition.

Manipulation and mobilisation

Manipulation is a forceful thrust in the desired direction. Mobilisation is a more gentle movement of the joints and tissues. Different disciplines approach manipulative therapy in different ways. Most physiotherapists use the Maitland Techniques which are effective for pain relief and for facilitating an improved range of movement. The treatment usually requires repeated visits, with detailed evaluation of the back at each session.

Chiropractic and osteopathy were devised by American bone-setters over the past century. The approach to treatment is to realign the spine and thus alleviate pain. Osteopaths and chiropractors base their treatment on the theory that they are putting displaced vertebrae back in place. Medical knowledge and science do not support this theory as it would require very strong forces to displace the vertebrae. Research has now shown that while some patients may well receive immediate relief from this type of spinal adjustment, this type of treatment may not have long-term benefits.

Alternative therapies

It may be useful to try alternative therapies such as acupuncture if other forms of recognised treatment have failed. Most will not do any harm. Like pain-killing drugs, however, they may give relief from pain but will not correct the underlying mechanical problem.

Reflexology is based on the belief that the body is divided into different zones which are represented on the toes and feet. A deep massage is applied to the area of the foot that represents the painful area of the body. Some patients get pain relief with this type of treatment. Reflexology has no scientific basis, but it is not harmful.

Exercise

Exercise plays a valuable part in reducing low back pain. The most appropriate type of exercise programme will depend on the individual back problem. Incorrect exercise or over-forceful exercise can do more harm than good. It is therefore important that exercise is carried out under careful professional supervision. Consult your physiotherapist prior to undertaking exercise.

There are two main categories of back exercise: mobilising exercises and strengthening exercises.

Mobilising exercises should be carried out when the range of movement in the spine has become stiff or limited. This can happen after prolonged periods of immobilisation or when adhesions have formed in the soft tissues as a result of injury. The two most common forms of mobilisation exercises are flexion (bending forward) and extension (bending back). It must be stressed that these movements must not be forced. Extension exercises such as standing upright and arching the back backwards can put large stresses on the lower lumbar spine. These types of exercise should only be carried out under supervision.

In general, most exercise programmes will be directed at strengthening the muscles. Strengthening exercises fall into two main categories: isometric and isotonic exercises.

Isometric exercises are usually prescribed during the acute stages of low back pain. They involve static contractions of the muscles, rather than movement of the spine itself, and are effective for maintaining muscle tone and strength during the acute stages.

Isotonic exercises are more intensive strengthening exercises which require movement of the spine. They will result in increasing the strength of the muscles throughout the range of movement. When adequate strength has been regained, these exercises can be done against the resistance of weights in order to strengthen the spine further. It is important that these exercises are carried out under professional supervision. Research has shown that strengthening of the abdominal and trunk muscles greatly assists in the control of chronic low back pain.

Hydrotherapy

Exercises in water can be effective once the acute pain has gone. The heat of the water, combined with gentle movement, can assist in controlling the problem. When swimming, use a gentle, easy stroke. The crawl and back-stroke are preferable. People with low back problems should not do the breast-stroke. Long-distance, easy swimming is more beneficial for the back.

Back braces or supports

It is not advisable to become dependent on back braces or supports as these tend to lead to stiffening of the spine. There are, however, cases in which they are useful in the acute stages of a low back problem. Back braces can also be useful for giving added support in work situations that necessitate heavy lifting.

WHAT IF CONSERVATIVE TREATMENT FAILS?

Should back pain persist after trying conservative treatment, the patient is then referred to an orthopaedic specialist for further investigation and treatment. Not all patients who require a specialist's opinion will require surgery. Operations are carried out only when absolutely necessary. Surgeons will give the patient the full facts about the pros and cons of surgery so the patient can decide whether he or she really wants to go on with surgical treatment. Other procedures that may be carried out by your consultant include epidurals and facet joint injections.

Epidurals are mainly carried out to stop acute episodes of pain. This is a way of anaesthetising the region to allow for full relief of pain and muscle spasm. The patient is admitted to hospital and confined to bed for a few days. The epidural space (the layer of fluid surrounding the spinal cord with the vertebral canal) is injected with drugs that have an anaesthetic effect on the back and lower limbs. The patient will feel immediate pain relief. After a few days of this type of treatment, the epidural is stopped. Patients report a marked improvement, and some report that they have complete relief from pain. This form of treatment is not suitable in all cases.

Injection into the facet joints (the small joints at either side of the back of the spine) is done under X-ray control with the use of dye. This type of technique has two purposes. It can give the patient good relief as the joints are injected with local anaesthetic and steroids. It is also used as a diagnostic procedure to assist in evaluating what joints are responsible for triggering the patient's pain.

SPINAL SURGERY

Discectomy or microdiscectomy

This is the most common form of spinal surgery. The objective of the operation is to remove protruded disc matter. This procedure is carried out for relief of leg pain (sciatica). It is never done for relief of back pain only. A small incision is made in the back and the surgeon exposes the nerve root that is being impinged on by the protruded disc matter. The majority of the disc is left behind and only the protruded matter is removed.

Nerve root/spinal decompression

An incision similar to that used for performing a discectomy is used to remove anything that is causing entrapment of one or more of the nerves within the lower lumbar spine. This usually involves removal of the excess bone produced by arthritis which is squeezing on a nerve root.

Spinal fusion

This surgical procedure joins together two or more unstable or painful vertebrae. A bone graft from the pelvis is usually used to provide the bony union. Sometimes metal fixation is also used to provide extra stabilisation. This is major spinal surgery and it is important that the bone graft is given every opportunity to fuse. To facilitate this, many activities are restricted for three to six months after the operation.

KEEPING YOUR BACK IN
GOOD CONDITION

If you have ever had back pain, or if you have just recovered from back problems, it is important to keep your back in good condition to avoid problems in the future. The main areas to take care of are posture, correct body mechanics and a healthy lifestyle.

When standing, sitting or lying, always remember that good posture will help to reduce the wear-and-tear forces on the back. When lifting, avoid stress on the back by following all the rules of lifting. Good body mechanics in relation to all activities of daily living – getting in and out of bed, standing from sitting – will protect your back. Keep your back straight when doing all physically strenuous tasks such as mowing the lawn, digging, hoovering, even ironing.

A healthy lifestyle, incorporating regular exercise, avoiding foods that put on excess weight, and reducing stress and tension can contribute significantly to building a healthy back.

If you have been given a programme of exercises by your physiotherapist, make the commitment to do them every day. If you have had a back problem, flexibility and strength in the muscles of the back are essential – weak back muscles increase your chances of further problems.

Mr Frank Dowling BSc, FRCSI is a Consultant Orthopaedic Surgeon at the Blackrock Clinic, Dublin, and Our Lady's Hospital for Sick Children, Crumlin. His speciality is the spine. **Marie Elaine Grant MISCP, MCSP** is Head of Physiotherapy at the Blackrock Clinic.

BEREAVEMENT – THE EXPERIENCE OF LOSS

THÉRÈSE BRADY

The days of keening over the coffin, wearing a black patch on your sleeve or retiring into widow's weeds are long gone. These traditional rituals of mourning have not been replaced, so that today, many of us have great difficulty in coping with bereavement, whether it is a personal loss or someone else's.

The study of how people react to bereavement is relatively new. Clinical psychologist Thérèse Brady unravels the complexities of the grieving process. This should be helpful to anyone who is trying to cope with the experience of loss or who has unresolved feelings of grief from the past. It may also help us be better prepared to deal with losses in the future . . .

Jenny, an only child, was eighteen months old when she died from cancer.

A month before John's retirement, his wife was diagnosed with a terminal illness. He had worked hard all his life. Both he and his wife had looked forward to his retirement and had planned to do many things they had not been able to do before. She died three months later.

David and Jane had been married for twenty-eight years when David left to live with another woman.

Mary was delighted when, at thirty-eight, she became pregnant for the first time. The baby was born with a severe mental handicap.

What do you say when you meet Jenny's parents – or John, Jane or Mary, all of whom have been bereaved? Do you say 'Sorry for your trouble' and depart? Do you avoid them altogether, or do you talk to them about what has happened?

Avoidance of the subject of loss of bereaved persons is common. This leaves the bereaved feeling isolated at a time when in greatest need of support. They feel that their grief is an unwelcome intrusion in the lives of others, that their presence is an embarrassment.

Why do we feel so uncomfortable when confronted with the distress of others, particularly when this concerns death and dying? There are many reasons.

As more people live longer and fewer people are part of a close-knit community, there is less direct experience of death and dying in the western world today than in the past. Experience of death and dying is more likely to come indirectly through the media. Death is remote; it happens elsewhere; it is often large-scale and unnatural, arising from war, famine or some other major disaster. Many will be more familiar with deaths in Somalia or Bosnia than in their own neighbourhood. As death has become increasingly distanced, dying has become more mechanised and professionalised, and is less likely to take place at home.

Unconscious fears of our own death or a conscious fear of the death of someone close to us also contribute to discomfort with death. The bereaved are a reminder that we too will be like them some day.

A major reason for distancing ourselves from the bereaved stems from a feeling of impotence. We don't know what to do or say. Even though we wish to alleviate the distress of the bereaved person, we are fearful that we may do or say the wrong thing. That fear is based on a false assumption that the pain of loss can be removed by the correct words or actions. Such an assumption fails to recognise the reality of the loss and denies the authenticity of the pain and sadness to which a major loss gives rise. Attempts to banish their pain by too hasty reassurances and efforts to distract them undermine the legitimacy of the distress of the bereaved. Grief needs time and space. It needs to be experienced and worked through.

Acknowledgment of their loss and of the legitimacy of their reactions is central to helping the bereaved. By having an understanding of the reactions to which a major loss gives rise, reactions at once universal yet unique to each individual, we can all be more supportive.

REACTIONS TO LOSS

People are frequently perplexed by reactions to loss. For the bereaved themselves, their reactions can be a source of concern. They wonder whether they are grieving in the proper way. They are acutely sensitive to the ways in which others are judging their grief. They may fear that they are going mad and or that they may disintegrate under the intensity of their grief. To realise that their reactions are normal can be a great relief. While reactions to loss are universal, not all of them will be experienced by all bereaved people nor experienced in the sequence described here. Some reactions will occur again and again. Bereavement cannot be neatly packaged in a time-limited, structured programme. It is a process that goes backwards and forwards at its own pace and in its own time.

When confronted with a major loss, be it a death, the diagnosis of a terminal illness or the birth of a handicapped child, the natural response is to seek protection from the reality of the loss by avoiding it or denying it. Sooner or later, the reality of the loss will penetrate the barriers set up as protection, bringing with it the pain to which loss inevitably gives rise. By confronting their loss and working through their grief, the bereaved will in time learn to adapt to a life without what has been lost. As a framework for understanding loss, reactions are described under three phases: the protective phase, the confrontation phase and the adaptation phase.

The protective phase: 'This is not happening to me'
The first response to traumatic news is frequently shock. Bereaved people commonly report that, following a death or the diagnosis of a terminal illness, they feel numb and dazed and function as automatons. They have a sense of depersonalisation, as if they were outsiders or onlookers at an event such as a funeral or burial that directly concerns them. Later, they may wonder how they continued to do the ordinary, everyday things. These reactions are powerful ways of protecting the system from being overwhelmed by the intensity of the trauma. They are often misunderstood, leading others to comment on how controlled the bereaved person is, on how well he or she is coping. Such remarks may be resented by the bereaved person because of the implication that she/he would appear more distressed if they really cared. Denial and disbelief that the loss has occurred may lead to rejection of a diagnosis of a terminal illness or a mental handicap. It is not uncommon for a bereaved person to wake up in the mornings as if from a bad dream, only to realise that the nightmare is a reality. These awakenings may recur over a long time. On each occasion, the bereaved person must confront afresh the stark reality of their loss.

Confronting the loss: 'This awful thing has happened and cannot be reversed'
As time goes on, the protective barrier of numbness,

depersonalisation and denial loses its effectiveness. The recognition of the irreversibility of the loss may then result in feelings of acute anxiety. Feelings of tightness in the chest, hyperventilation and other psychosomatic sensations may increase anxiety feelings to a level of panic. The bereaved may believe that they have the same symptoms as those of the person who died and that their own death is now imminent. They may feel confused and disorganised, unable to make even simple decisions such as what clothes to wear. They may be frightened about their ability to cope. These symptoms can be so overwhelming that they lead the bereaved to feel that they are losing control and going mad. Learning that these symptoms are normal following bereavement is reassuring, that they stem from anxiety about a future in a world that no longer seems safe or predictable.

Wrenching pangs of grief are common. The bereaved person may feel that his/her body is being physically torn apart. Tears may come in floods or may be suppressed, for we have learned so well in childhood that 'big boys/girls do not cry'. Crying, which can provide such a healthy emotional release, is an embarrassment to all. The bereaved will pine and yearn for what has been lost. They may wish to go back in time and to change something in the sequence of events that could have resulted in a different outcome. '*O call back yesterday, bid time return*' (Shakespeare, *Richard II*). The mother would not have sent her child on that message which led to his death in a traffic accident; the husband would have told his wife how much he loved her. The longing to have the deceased back may lead the bereaved to search for them. They may call out to them or may follow someone in a crowd, believing it to be the deceased. They may hear the voice or the footsteps of their loved one and run to open the door to them, only to be constantly disappointed. They will continue to consult them. All these reactions are normal. The loss of someone's physical presence does not result in the loss of the experience of them.

A major loss may result in strong feelings of anger – anger

against the doctor who failed to prevent the death or who did not care for the deceased and their surviving relatives as the bereaved would have wished; anger against God, against relatives who were not there when needed. The anger may be directed against the person who has gone, leaving the bereaved to cope with the distressful consequences of their departure, for example, with the guilt and shame that follow on a suicide. Such negative emotions may be upsetting, for how can you feel angry with someone who has died, with someone you loved? The co-existence of conflicting emotions such as sadness and relief, love and anger, which are normal, is an added source of distress.

Feelings of regret, remorse and guilt are common. The bereaved will ruminate about the many things that they did or did not do or say. The daughter who looked after a demanding mother for years will feel guilty about the times she resented her or wished her dead; the father will regret his harshness towards his son. There is now no opportunity of putting things right. While there may be remorse and guilt over normal human failings, guilt can also arise in the context of real errors. For example, the bereaved may have caused the death by driving when drunk. The expression of guilt is frequently blocked by others who, uncomfortable with such expressions, rush to reassure the bereaved that they have no cause to feel guilty. Yet the bereaved need to express these feelings and to have them accepted.

While blaming themselves for their failings, the bereaved may idealise the deceased. The husband, known to have given his wife a difficult time, is described as having been kind and caring; the dead child is remembered as a saint. Remarks that the child 'was too good for this world' encourage such sanctification and can result in the unfavourable comparison of surviving children with the child who has died. 'Why weren't you the one to die?' asked a mother, deeply missing the child who has died and now exasperated by her six-year-old.

Among the most painful emotions experienced by bereaved people are feelings of hopelessness, futility and despair. What has John to live for after the death of his wife to whom he had been married for forty-five years? Recently retired, his family has long since left home; no one has need of him any longer. Or Patricia, who devoted the last fifteen years to the care of her only child, born with a severe physical disability. She too can see little purpose in living. This sense of hopelessness and despair can be overwhelming, both for the bereaved and for those who would wish to console them.

The loneliness that follows a loss can be acute, a loneliness experienced as much when surrounded by others as in the emptiness of the home. While the empty place at the table or in the bed, or the missing of a partner or friend in whom to confide, constantly reinforce the feelings of loneliness, the sense of being on one's own, bereft of child, parent or spouse, can be at its most painful in the midst of a crowd.

Trying to make sense of what has happened can lead to ceaseless questioning. How could an all-powerful and merciful God allow a child or the mother of a young family to die? Why did this happen to me? Is there a life after death? These questions may be pursued endlessly without finding any satisfactory answer.

Learning to live with the loss: Life must go on
Unimaginable as it may have seemed at one time, the bereaved do come through the awfulness of their grief. While some may never 'get over it', the pain of loss becomes less intense and less frequent. Preoccupation with what has been lost will lessen. Pangs of grief, triggered by sudden memories, will still occur, often when least expected. There can be a fear of forgetting the person who has died, what they looked like, how their voice sounded. Yet, while those images fade, the memories remain. 'Since I stopped bothering about it,' writes C S Lewis, referring to fear of losing the memory of his deceased wife, 'she seems to meet me everywhere.' Adjustment to life without what has been lost calls for adaptation and change. The role filled by a father will be taken over in part by other members of the family; the

mother will have to reorder a day previously built around the needs of her sick child.

Mourning is seen as a duty to the dead. Today it is difficult to know when that duty has been fulfilled. When is it appropriate to resume 'normal' life, to go to the pub, to enjoy oneself, to start a new relationship? Rituals that existed in the past, such as wearing black for a specified length of time, provided a socially sanctioned way of beginning and ending grief. With time, the bereaved learn to let go of the mourning without feeling guilty. They adapt to a world that is changed by virtue of what has been lost and gradually shift their emotional energy from a concern with what has been lost to the development of a new and adaptive life without the deceased. Such adaptation is a continuing process which may take one or several years, depending on the nature and consequences of the loss.

THE UNIQUENESS OF EACH LOSS

While sharing with other bereaved persons some or all of the usual reactions to loss, the experience of loss is different for each individual. The response to loss will be influenced by the nature of the loss, by personal characteristics, previous experiences and coping strategies, by the meaning and consequences of the loss, and by the resources available to deal with the loss.

THE NATURE AND CIRCUMSTANCES
OF THE LOSS

The nature of the loss, be it death, marital separation, infertility or loss of physical functioning, will influence the response to the loss. When the loss arises through death, the nature and circumstances of the death, whether resulting from an accident, a suicide or a prolonged illness, will have important implications. Violent deaths, including accidents, suicide and homicide, are the major cause of death in those under forty years of age. Adjustment to such deaths is particularly difficult. The initial shock and subsequent grief reactions may be more intense and prolonged. The lack of preparation for the death, the abruptness of change, the circumstances and consequences of the death, all contribute to the difficulties experienced. Was the bereaved there at the time of the death? If not, how did they learn about it? Did the death lead to inquests and court proceedings?

In general, adjustment to death anticipated because of age or illness is less difficult. There is time to prepare for the death, opportunities to share love and forgiveness, to plan for life after the death. To be able to do so is helpful for both the person who is dying and for those left to grieve. But such communication is not always possible. The person who is dying and their loved ones may derive comfort from the belief that, by not talking about the impending death, they are protecting each other. While allowing time for preparation, the potential impact of anticipated deaths should not be underestimated.

Caring for a loved one over a prolonged and often unpredictable course may leave the bereaved physically and emotionally drained. Feelings of relief that the dead person's suffering and/or that the burden of caring for them is over may co-exist with great sadness. When the care of a chronically or terminally ill person has been the main preoccupation, the vacuum left by the death will be great. Nor should the potential impact of the death of an elderly parent be lightly dismissed. That someone has had 'a good innings' does not take from the fact that a parent who has always been part of your life will no longer be there.

The way in which a person dies is important. Great comfort can be derived from a death that was peaceful and dignified and at which the bereaved was present. In contrast, deaths arising from suicide or AIDS are particularly difficult to cope with because of the stigma, the added sense of blame, of failure, of isolation that all too frequently accompany them.

CHARACTERISTICS OF THE BEREAVED

The bereaved should not be stereotyped into a single category. Each bereaved person will continue to be more like his or her distinctive self than like other persons similarly bereaved. Some may be reserved, less likely to express their emotions openly or to want to talk about their concerns; others may cry readily and talk continually about their loss. The response to loss will be in a style characteristic to each individual. It will also be influenced by experiences of previous losses or other stressful events. A relatively small loss may trigger other losses, resulting in what appears greater upset for this small loss than for a previous major loss. Those with a dependent type of personality may have particular difficulty in coping, such is their sense of helplessness in facing the future without the deceased.

The relationship with what has been lost and the meaning of that loss are important. The death of a husband may mean the loss of the breadwinner, the social and sexual partner, the handyman and the confidant. The death of a child may mean the loss of the mother's primary role. The bereaved, much of whose role stemmed from their unique relationship with the deceased, will lose a significant part of themselves. The quality of the relationship with the deceased is also important. Where that relationship has been good, the bereaved, while missing the deceased very much, can fall back on the security of that relationship and on good memories of shared experiences. A conflictual relationship on the other hand may leave the bereaved with a sense of unfinished business and resentment towards the partner who has left him/her to cope with the additional burdens arising from the death.

Age, both of the person who has died as well as of the bereaved, should be considered too. All too frequently, the impact of a loss on older adults or on children is underestimated.

Older adults, who may have little to look forward to, and who have to adjust to living on their own for the first time, may find little reason to go on living. If a son or daughter dies before them, they may feel guilty.

Children are frequently excluded from the events surrounding a death because they are considered too young to understand or too vulnerable because of their immaturity. Yet even very young children are affected by a major loss. Their understanding of the loss will be influenced by their level of intellectual development. Thus the young child is unable to grasp the irreversibility of death. 'Is Grandpa still dead today?' asked the novelist Georges Sand, at the age of four, the day after her grandfather's death. Young children are egocentric. They tend to perceive whatever happens as a consequence of their own thoughts and actions. In a fit of pique, a child may wish its mother dead and may then assume the blame for that death should the mother subsequently die. The child links good and bad outcomes to its own behaviour. Death is therefore not fortuitous. It is a punishment for bad behaviour. Adults unwittingly foster such beliefs with comments such as 'You must be very good if you want your daddy to get better', even though the child's behaviour and the father's illness are totally unconnected. If the father dies, the child may assume blame and try by good behaviour to bring the father back again. The child's thinking is also concrete in nature. They may be concerned about the dead person feeling hungry, cold or lonely. A six-year-old wanted his mother to put on the electric blanket 'to warm Granny up'. It is not until the child is about nine that the concept of death as biological, inevitable and irreversible is grasped.

Children's reactions to loss are often masked. They may regress and start to bed-wet or soil. They may become excessively clinging. The death of one parent may lead to intense anxiety that the other parent too may die. Problems in eating and sleeping, physical symptoms such as pains and aches as well as behavioural problems, particularly in teenagers, are common. The quality of school work may fall off. The reason for this behaviour is frequently misunderstood and often results in punishment. The child is left to feel isolated, rejected and guilty.

THE CONSEQUENCES OF LOSS

While the nature and significance of the loss and the characteristics of the bereaved are important determinants of the response to loss, so too are the consequences of the loss, which may be physical, emotional, social, material and/or spiritual in nature.

Physical symptoms such as insomnia, loss of appetite and tiredness are common. Stress heightens vulnerability to physical illness and disease. Bereavement is associated with an increase in physical symptoms, in visits to the doctor and in mortality rates.

The intensity of the emotions that follow a major loss may leave the bereaved emotionally drained. While some are concerned about feeling dead inside and their inability to feel anything, others are overwhelmed by emotions such as anxiety, anger or guilt. Feelings of depression and despair leave one depleted of energy. 'No one ever told me about the laziness of grief,' writes C S Lewis. 'I loathe the slightest effort.'

Socially, the bereaved frequently feel isolated and shunned. In the days and weeks following a death, there are usually many callers, letters and other demonstrations of concern. With time, these diminish. The bereaved person is left to get on with life, in the mistaken belief that the greatest distress occurs at the time of the death itself. This is not so. It may be weeks or months before the reality of the loss impinges. The withdrawal of social support may leave the individual feeling doubly bereft. The person who has derived much of their role and status from the deceased may find themselves particularly at a loss. Those who have lost a partner frequently feel stigmatised. Society can make it difficult for widows or widowers to join in social activities. For the child too, the absence of a parent because of death or separation can be a source of embarrassment .

A major loss frequently has serious material and practical consequences. For example, the death of a father may result in the loss of income, the loss of a car or even of the family home, and may leave the mother to combine the roles of breadwinner and homemaker. She must take on added responsibilities, perhaps including work outside the home, at a time when her own personal resources are so depleted. Where a mother dies leaving young children, arrangements must be made for their care. Some families may be able to fall back on relatives; others will have to employ a carer. This can lead to an additional financial burden, as well as to resentment on the part of the children towards someone taking on the role of their mother. Some widowers try to look after the home themselves, undertaking domestic tasks such as cooking and washing, perhaps for the first time. Fulfilling the double role of breadwinner and homemaker makes heavy demands on time, leaving the surviving partner little time for themselves and at risk of increased isolation. The death of a parent also impacts on the role of the children, often leaving them to take on additional responsibilities. The eldest daughter may step into the shoes of her mother or the eldest boy into those of his father, looking after the younger children and acting as companion and confidant for the surviving parent. This can be a heavy burden for a young person.

Loss may also have spiritual consequences. Death raises fundamental issues. What is life all about? Is there a life after death? For some, belief in God and in an afterlife is a source of consolation. For others, a major loss calls these beliefs into question. They feel let down by God, and may find it difficult to maintain their faith. They need to struggle with the issues of life and death in their own way and should not be expected to respond readily to the firm convictions of others.

HELPING THE BEREAVED

Learning to live with loss requires time, an acknowledgement of the reality of the loss, and experiencing the pain of that loss. Grief cannot be hurried. Its onset may be delayed, but sooner or later the bereaved person must give in to the pain in order to come through their grief. A bereaved person may never get over his or her loss, but can learn to move forward in a world changed because of that loss. While others cannot take the pain of loss away, they can help by providing support, understanding and security. Support lets the bereaved person know that there are people on whom they can call. Understanding brings with it an acceptance of the bereaved person as he or she is. Security provides a sense of safety in facing a changed and unpredictable world.

A respect for each person's loss and individual style of grieving, together with a sensitivity to the particular needs of that individual, are key elements in the support of the bereaved. For those wishing to help, it may mean listening to the same story over and over again. Reviewing the death and the events leading up to it, as well as one's life with the deceased, are often helpful ways of coming to terms with the loss. Losses should not be minimised. Feelings should be legitimised. Bereaved individuals should not be made to feel guilty for continuing to grieve. They may seem self-centred at times, and the would-be supporters discouraged and even irritated by the bereaved person's failure to reward them by responding positively to their efforts. The expectations that others have of how bereaved persons should grieve can impact on an already poor self-esteem by making the bereaved feel that they are failing to 'grieve properly' and are therefore nuisances to everyone.

A sensitivity to the physical, social, sexual, spiritual and practical as well as to the emotional needs of the bereaved will indicate important ways of providing support. Different people can help in different ways. At times, a small gesture such as dropping in an apple tart or taking the children out for a couple of hours may be particularly appreciated. Support should not mean crowding out the bereaved, for example, by arranging a 24-hour rota to ensure that mother is never left on her own. The bereaved need time and space to grieve on their own and to learn that they can come to live without what has been lost. It can often be difficult to get the balance right between offering too much or too little support. And indeed, at times, nothing seems to help. When unsure of what to do, it is best to check with the bereaved. Indeed, it is helpful if the bereaved take the initiative by indicating what their needs are and how they can be helped. Sometimes, support can come from family and friends; at other times it will come from outside their personal network, from the teachers at school, from neighbours whom they had scarcely known before the death, or from others who have been similarly bereaved. Bereavement support groups are now available in some parts of the country. They can provide a useful source of understanding and support for those who feel that their own family and friends are tiring of them and of their expressions of grief. A small number of bereaved individuals experiencing particular difficulty with grieving may need professional help. There are now many useful books on grieving for both adults and children. Bereaved people derive much reassurance by learning from such literature that their own reactions are quite normal.

The year immediately following the loss is full of first anniversaries. Some, such as birthdays and Christmas, are anticipated with apprehension. Others, such as the day 'he went into hospital', may not, but can still be equally distressing. Some feel freer to move forward once they have completed a cycle of anniversaries. For others, it takes longer to let go of grieving for what has been lost and to replace lost hopes, plans and relationships with new ones.

Loss is an integral part of life; bereavement, an integral part of love. We grow through love, but also through suffering. For the bereaved, that growth, the discovery of new strengths and capacities, is nurtured by the acceptance and understanding of others, and by their affirmation of the bereaved as they are, and not as they might wish them to be.

Only people who are capable of loving strongly can also suffer great sorrow, but this same necessity of loving serves to counteract their grief and heal them.

Tolstoy

Thérèse Brady FPsSI, FIHF is Director of the Postgraduate Programme in Clinical Psychology at University College, Dublin. She is responsible for the development of Volunteer Bereavement Services at Our Lady's Hospice and St Francis Hospice, Dublin.

BOWEL PROBLEMS

PROFESSOR WILLIAM KIRWAN

Bowel problems affect all of us at some time. These problems vary in severity. We may get an occasional dose of diarrhoea from exam nerves or a bout of 'Delhi Belly' on holiday, or we may find life dominated by a chronic condition such as Crohn's disease or colitis.

Professor of Surgery William Kirwan deals here with a wide range of bowel problems, from the relatively minor irritable bowel syndrome to the most serious condition, bowel cancer . . .

The bowel as a whole consists of the small bowel above and the large bowel below. The function of the small bowel is the absorption of food and it is therefore of great importance in nutrition. The function of the large bowel is the absorption of water and the storage of waste for elimination at a convenient time. The large bowel is again divided into the colon above and the rectum below. In general, nature has provided us with a large reserve of bowel. A person can function satisfactorily even after a considerable length of bowel has been lost due to surgery or disease.

When food is swallowed, digestion begins in the stomach. Partly digested food is passed gradually out of the stomach into the small bowel. As it passes down the length of the small bowel, nutrition is extracted from it. By the time it reaches the large bowel, it consists only of residue and water. In its passage through the large bowel, the water is absorbed and the residue is concentrated into a solid which is passed out as stool.

Frequency of bowel movements is extremely variable from person to person. Two motions per day might be normal for one person, while one motion every two days may be normal for another. Most people have a clearly established bowel habit. It is a change in the habit, rather than the habit itself, that is important.

BOWEL CONDITIONS

Irritable bowel syndrome

This is extremely common and is not dangerous. It results from a spasm of the bowel and may be related to a deficiency of dietary fibre. The entire gut has very complex nerve connections with the central nervous system. There are many conditions such as migraine that are triggered by stress, and irritable bowel syndrome is also probably in this category. It is probable that stress perceived by the brain is transmitted unconsciously to the bowel, resulting in the bowel behaviour that constitutes irritable bowel syndrome. The bowel behaves erratically and can fluctuate between constipation and diarrhoea. There is often some lower

78

abdominal discomfort, particularly on the left side. X-rays of the bowel will reveal no significant abnormality but are often necessary to rule out serious disease. This is one of the most common bowel complaints that causes patients to consult their doctors. Irritable bowel syndrome is an unsatisfactory and very improvised name for not a single but probably a group of conditions that are poorly understood.

Gastroenteritis

This has also been called 'traveller's diarrhoea'. It is related to dietary changes and also to the consumption of contaminated food.

The most fundamental item of diet is water. If you travel, find out whether the water is safe. In hot countries where water may be unsafe, avoid ice and use bottled water. Seek advice from those who have already visited the place, as they will advise you about what to avoid. Always take an anti-diarrhoea preparation with you when you travel. Excellent and safe examples are Lomotil and Imodium. If you get diarrhoea, drink clear liquids for twenty-four hours and the problem will usually settle. It is unlikely that you will have to consult a doctor. If the problem persists after your return, however, you should see your family doctor.

Piles (haemorrhoids)

Piles are extremely common. They consist of clusters of tissue, containing a lot of blood vessels, just inside the anal region. They may come down on emptying the bowel, particularly if there is straining. At this time, due to the straining, they become injured and bleed. The blood is bright red in colour and sometimes squirts out alarmingly. The patient will often feel something coming down which goes back afterwards. In more advanced cases, however, the piles may stay down permanently. Piles can be very troublesome during pregnancy, although they will often regress, but not disappear, following delivery.

Piles are treated by the simplest method possible, reserving

79

surgery for the more severe cases. The most common cause of piles is some degree of constipation, so correcting this with a high-fibre diet is often sufficient. Over-the-counter preparations may help the patient through periods of discomfort while the diet is being corrected, but such preparations treat the effect and not the cause and do not provide a permanent solution to the problem. It is generally undesirable for patients to treat themselves with over-the-counter preparations in the absence of a diagnosis. If symptoms persist for two weeks, they should consult the family doctor. Surgery for severe cases gives excellent results, but it is again emphasised that the majority of cases can be treated by diet alone.

A diagnosis of haemorrhoids must be made by a doctor who will examine the patient and eliminate more serious possibilities. Patients must not neglect rectal symptoms in the belief that they are due to haemorrhoids. Severe anal pain is unlikely to be due to haemorrhoids and is often caused by an anal fissure (a crack in the very sensitive skin of the anal canal). This distressing condition responds well to surgery.

Crohn's disease

This is an inflammation which can affect any part of the bowel but which is more troublesome when it affects the small bowel. It results in diarrhoea and crampy pain, as the bowel is narrowed and food has difficulty getting through. This results in pain after eating. The cause is unknown, although it predominantly affects young people. Patients are treated with drugs unless problems are severe. If this treatment fails, usually due to extreme narrowing of the bowel, the damaged part of the intestine may have to be removed surgically. Crohn's disease has a bad reputation for recurrence following surgery, but this is in fact not justified. The majority of patients get good results from surgery and enjoy an excellent quality of life. A small minority, however, have continuing significant problems.

Ulcerative colitis

This is frequently referred to by patients simply as colitis. It is an inflammation of the colon and rectum of unknown cause. It has some resemblance to Crohn's disease but its management is quite different. The main symptom is bloody diarrhoea. This can vary greatly in severity from once or twice per day to more than twenty times per day. The patient loses a lot of water, minerals and blood and becomes dehydrated, weak and anaemic. Patients, who are often in their teens, twenties or thirties, feel threatened by incontinence when out and about and will worry about the availability of toilet facilities. This tends to restrict the mobility and independence of such patients, and normal functions like shopping or attending church may become the cause of great anxiety or may even become impossible.

Patients are treated medically, often with steroids and other drugs, and a great many are controlled by these methods. Continuing severe diarrhoea, however, may make life impossible and such patients are offered surgery. Traditional surgery, which gave excellent results, involved removal of the entire bowel, leaving the patient with a permanent ileostomy (a bag, see 'Stomas', page 84). In recent years, there has been considerable progress in preserving the lower part of the patient's bowel, and the construction of a pouch reservoir in the pelvis to replace the removed bowel. This new operation gives good results, but there is a failure rate of approximately 10 per cent. The operation, however, is very attractive for young patients who, understandably, wish to avoid an ileostomy.

Diverticular disease

Diverticular disease (diverticulosis) is extremely common in western society and is related to the consumption of a diet high in refined carbohydrate and low in dietary fibre. The condition is extremely rare in those countries where the staple diet consists mainly of vegetable material containing much fibre. In this condition, the pressure in the bowel is abnormally high, and this results in small bulges or blow-outs in the wall of the bowel. These are like little sacs attached to the outside of the bowel. Lodgment of material in these sacs can result in complications.

Most middle-aged people in Ireland have these abnormal pouches in their colon, and in fact they rarely cause trouble. A number of patients, however, may complain of pain in the left lower abdomen due to spasm of the bowel. A smaller number again may get acute inflammation (diverticulitis) and these may require hospitalisation and intensive treatment.

The treatment of this condition is improvement of the diet, increasing the amount of fibre. The ideal source of fibre is bran, and the patient should gradually work up towards a dose of two tablespoonsful per day. This usually gets rid of symptoms and improves bowel action.

It is emphasised that the presence of this condition in itself is of little significance and problems will not arise if the patient takes sufficient fibre.

Polyps

Polyps are like grapes hanging on a stalk inside the bowel. They usually result in the passage of blood. Polyps can become malignant and should therefore be removed. This can be done by passing an instrument into the bowel from below. A person who has had a polyp may develop further polyps in the future and will therefore require continuing follow-up by his or her doctor.

Bowel cancer

Bowel cancer arises in the colon and rectum. It is the most common serious form of cancer in Ireland in males who do not smoke (lung cancer is more common in smokers). Bowel cancer comes second to breast cancer in females, but with increased smoking, this order is likely to be reversed. Patients with bowel cancer usually have a change in bowel habit and often pass blood. Anaemia is another common presentation.

Disturbance of bowel habit is extremely common due to ordinary events in life such as gastroenteritis, but if it persists for two weeks, the family doctor should be consulted. In many instances, doctors will be able to satisfy themselves that there is no serious problem. They may decide to observe the patient for a further period during which the symptoms may disappear completely. If symptoms persist, however, further investigation is required.

Bowel cancer is curable if diagnosed early. Surgery is the only really effective treatment. Other types of treatment, which are effective in different types of cancer, have little fundamental effect on bowel cancer. Surgery consists of removing a length of diseased bowel and joining up the ends. In most cases (but not in all), it is unnecessary for the patient to have a colostomy (a bag, see 'Stomas', page 84).

A family history of bowel cancer can be important. It is probably only significant, however, if at least two close relatives have had the disease. Many people have somebody in their extended family who has had bowel cancer, but this should not cause particular anxiety.

Incontinence

This is a subject that people are reluctant to discuss and many who suffer from it consider that they are, in fact, unique. It has emerged, however, that the condition is quite common, affecting females almost entirely, particularly those who have had babies delivered by normal methods. It is now known that normal delivery may be associated with a downward pulling on important nerves in the pelvis, resulting in damage and subsequent muscle weakness. This is more likely to occur if a woman has had several babies. Problems with the bowel rarely come on immediately, but a number of women, at approximately the age of fifty, begin to notice poor bowel control. In certain cases, this can go on to cause severe problems. This problem has only recently been recognised. Procedures to correct it are being developed but are still quite imperfect. Women who suffer from this problem should realise that they are by no means unique and should seek the advice of their doctors.

Constipation

Most cases of constipation are due to poor diet and can be managed by increasing the intake of dietary fibre. There is, however, a group of young women who, in spite of a satisfactory diet, are severely constipated. The cause of the problem in this specific group is poorly understood and in addition to high-fibre intake, some will require laxatives. Laxatives in general are undesirable and should be used only as a last resort. Many preparations are available over-the-counter but it is more desirable for patients to consult a doctor before any treatment.

Stomas (ileostomy, colostomy)

Patients frequently refer to this as 'the bag'. In some cases of colitis, Crohn's disease or cancer, it is possible to remove the diseased part of the digestive tract and join the two ends together again. In other cases, it may be necessary to make an opening in the abdomen called a stoma, through which waste material can pass into a lightweight bag which is attached to the skin. Excellent stoma equipment is now available, and stoma-care departments exist in major hospitals, where special staff are available to advise and help. Patients with stomas should have a normal life. They work in every trade and profession, marry, have babies and quickly adapt to their new situation without difficulty. With modern methods and equipment, these patients rarely have to seek medical advice and in fact come to consider themselves as entirely normal. A stoma is a price that occasionally has to be paid for cure, but is in fact rarely a problem in itself.

DIETARY FIBRE

Dietary fibre (also referred to as roughage) consists of vegetable material that is not digested in the bowel and is passed out unaltered. Water adheres to the fibre, making the bowel content softer. It is therefore more easily propelled through the bowel and eliminated without straining. People vary in their requirements for dietary fibre. It is often mistakenly believed that fruit contains a large amount of fibre. In fact, an apple or orange is more than 90 per cent water. By comparison, bran contains 90 per cent dry fibrous material and is by far the best way to improve bowel function. It is, of course, rather dull and patients require some determination to take it regularly. Many breakfast cereals contain significant amounts of fibre.

If the nation consumed more dietary fibre, it is likely that there would be a much lower incidence of bowel cancer, diverticular disease, irritable bowel syndrome, haemorrhoids, appendicitis and many other disorders. In this area, therefore, much more can be achieved by common-sense diet than by expensive medical interventions.

BOWEL TESTS

Barium enema – This is an X-ray in which material is passed through a tube into the bowel so that the radiologist can see it. The bowel must be carefully emptied in advance. It is usually an out-patient procedure.

Sigmoidoscopy – The doctor passes an instrument into the bowel to examine the lower part. Much significant disease is within reach of this instrument. This is an out-patient procedure.

Colonoscopy – The patient is given a sedative drug and a long flexible instrument is passed in from below to examine the entire large bowel. The bowel must be carefully emptied beforehand. The procedure gives a precise view of the bowel, usually displayed on a television monitor. This is a day-case procedure.

DANGER SIGNALS

A doctor should be consulted for the following symptoms:
• Recent persistent change in bowel habit.
• A frequent desire to evacuate the bowel with unsatisfactory results.
• The passage of blood.
• Recent persisting abdominal cramps.

William Kirwan MCH, FRCS is Professor of Surgery at University College, Cork, and a Consultant Surgeon at Cork Regional Hospital.

BREAST CANCER

PROFESSOR NIALL O'HIGGINS

Approximately one in thirteen women in Ireland develops breast cancer, but the disease is treatable if caught early. Women are encouraged to see their doctor as soon as they suspect there is something unusual happening to their breast.

Professor Niall O'Higgins, a surgeon with a particular interest in breast cancer, explains what these changes are, the risk factors associated with the disease, and the different therapies used in treating breast cancer today . . .

Cancer is a global problem. It represents a significant threat to health and life all over the world, but is particularly evident in economically developed and industrialised countries such as those of the European Community (EC) where a high proportion of the population is elderly and therefore has a greater risk of cancer. In spite of progress in understanding the basis of cancer and of increasingly successful treatments for some of its forms, cancer remains one of the most feared group of diseases in the world. Quite appropriately, much of the fear is due to the fact that there is no cure for many types of cancer at present. Other fears, however, such as the belief that cancer and its treatment are invariably painful, distressing and associated with severe long-term suffering are quite misplaced. Some cancers are undoubtedly curable. Even for those that are not, effective control of pain and other distressing symptoms should be available to all patients.

Cancer is a group of diseases that occur when the cells of the organ or part of the body grow and proliferate in a disorderly, uncontrolled fashion. These uncontrolled cancer cells fulfil no useful function, and as they grow, they tend to replace the normal cells of the organ in which they develop and so interfere with the function of that organ. Some cells break away and are swept into the bloodstream to other parts of the body where they may lodge, start to grow in number and continue their destructive process. Such breakaway cells that settle and grow in other organs are called secondaries or metastases.

THE PROBLEM OF BREAST CANCER

Breast cancer is an important public health issue. It is the most common cancer among women in the EC where an estimated 135,000 new cases and 58,000 recorded deaths are reported per year. It is responsible for 24 per cent of all cancers and 18 per cent of all cancer deaths. The table in the Appendix shows the incidence of breast cancer among women in the EC. The incidence rate ranges between 39 per 100,000 in Spain to 75 per 100,000 in Ireland.

The reasons for the variation between northern and southern

Europe are unknown, but major research is being carried out to investigate whether these differences could be related to diet, alcohol and lifestyle factors. Ireland is closely involved in this large study, together with researchers from fifteen other countries.

RISK FACTORS FOR BREAST CANCER

Breast cancer is rare under the age of thirty. Thereafter, there is a steady rise in incidence up to the age of about forty-five. Between forty-five and fifty-five, the incidence is fairly static. It rises again up to the age of eighty. A woman's family history represents a risk factor; the daughter of a woman with breast cancer has a two- to three-fold risk of developing the disease herself. This risk is much greater in someone whose mother developed breast cancer at a young age. Pregnancy at an early age confers some degree of protection against the development of breast cancer. Women who have had many children are less likely to develop the disease than those who have not borne children. There also appears to be a slightly increased risk in women who had their first period at an early age and a late menopause, when compared with those who had the first period at a relatively late age and an early menopause. Some relatively unusual types of benign breast conditions may put the patient at a slightly increased risk for breast cancer, but in general benign breast conditions do not predispose to cancer development. Breast cancer is neither contagious nor infectious.

BREAST PAIN

The breast is under the influence of internal hormones or chemicals that are released from other glands of the body such as the ovaries, adrenals, thyroid and pituitary glands. The effects of these hormones on the breast vary from day to day during the menstrual cycle, and even from morning to evening within the same day. It is not surprising, therefore, that the texture and size of the breast varies during the menstrual cycle and that discomfort or even pain is experienced, particularly in the latter half of the cycle. This type of cyclical discomfort is common, although its mechanism is not fully understood. Most women with this condition can be helped by a full medical examination which usually provides the reassurance that there is no serious problem. For women with persistent pain, effective medications are available, although these should be used rather sparingly because they are often associated with unpleasant side-effects.

THE DETECTION OF BREAST CANCER

Although there are some exceptions, the outlook for patients with breast cancer is directly related to the size of the tumour or lump at the time of treatment. Thus patients with large tumours tend to have a less favourable outlook than those with smaller tumours. Patients with tiny tumours do best of all. All tumours start as small abnormalities, so it makes sense to find the cancer as early as possible, since the long-term outlook is likely to be so much better.

Breast self-examination

In the past, breast self-examination was advocated widely by public education media, cancer societies and health promotion agencies. This advice was based on the belief that tumours found on breast self-examination were likely to be smaller than those found accidentally. In general, the smaller the tumour is at the time of treatment, the better is the long-term outlook for the patient. Unfortunately, it has not been positively proven that tumours found on purposeful breast self-examination are smaller than those found fortuitously. There is insufficient evidence to support the theory that breast self-examination improves survival. It is a relatively insensitive method of breast examination when compared with physical examination by a doctor and mammography. For these reasons, general advice to the public about the value of breast self-examination in improving cure rates is no longer recommended. However, individual tuition and counselling by specialist nurses about breast self-examination is certainly to be encouraged because it helps a woman understand the normal changes that occur in her breasts. When carefully done, it avoids the excessive anxiety that occurs among some women when breast self-examination is advocated through the public media networks.

Signs and symptoms of breast cancer

Every woman should be encouraged to understand the changes occurring within the breasts throughout the monthly cycle. In this way, identification of any new development or change will be appreciated.

• A lump in the breast is often easily identified and should always be reported. Most lumps in the breast are quite innocent. Breast cancer lumps are generally hard and the texture of the lump is quite different from the surrounding tissue.

• A dimpling or depression in the skin, any change in contour, or any recent indrawing of the nipple should be reported to the doctor immediately, as these are all signs associated with breast cancer.

• Any bleeding from the nipple or persistent discharge, particularly if only on one side, should also be reported.

• A sore on the surface of the breast or nipple that does not heal may be an indicator of early cancer.

• Persistent breast pain or discomfort that occurs on one breast only and that is not related to the menstrual cycle should also be investigated.

• Enlarged, firm or hard glands or lumps in the armpit or neck sometimes indicate a breast tumour.

Mammography

A mammogram is an X-ray of the breast. In recent years, the quality of mammography has improved to the extent where small tumours are now frequently detected by mammogram alone long before any abnormality is discovered on clinical (physical) examination. Many of the tiny tumours found on mammography can now be cured without removing the breast. Another important technical point about modern mammography is that the dose of radiation per examination is now much lower than it was in the 1970s and early 1980s, thus making the examination safer.

The procedure involves two or three films on each breast. It is often an uncomfortable examination because, in order to obtain the best image, the breast is compressed or squeezed. A film is then taken from above and another from the side.

Limitations of mammography

Although modern mammography can give excellent definition of breast abnormalities, mammograms still miss from 10 to 15 per cent of cancers. Some of these cancers could well be discovered by careful clinical examination. Screening procedures should therefore not be restricted to mammograms but should combine mammography with clinical examination. Mammograms are of little or no value in very young women and in general are not recommended for women under the age of forty. This is because the breast tissue of young women is dense, so the discriminating value of a mammogram in detecting an abnormality is limited. Other investigations, such as ultrasound examination, are sometimes of value in the younger patient.

Who should have a mammogram?

All women aged fifty and over should have a mammogram and clinical examination, and this should be repeated every two to three years. Those with a family history of breast cancer or who have a history of breast abnormality should have their first mammogram at the age of forty. Any woman with a suspected breast cancer should have a mammogram to check on the opposite breast and to make sure that there is not a second tumour present.

THE TREATMENT OF BREAST CANCER

The treatment and outlook of patients with breast cancer depend on the type of tumour and the stage of the disease. Breast cancer is not a single condition and represents a wide variety of different types of disorders. The primary treatment involves consideration of four kinds of therapy: surgery, radiotherapy, chemotherapy and hormonal therapy. These treatments are given either singly or in combination, depending on the circumstances.

Surgery

In general, patients with breast cancer are now presenting with smaller tumours than was the case even ten years ago. For smaller tumours, particularly those near the periphery of the breast, mastectomy (removal of the breast) may not be needed. Many such tumours can be treated by quadrantectomy, which means the removal of the segment of the breast containing the tumour. The surgeon will normally remove a margin of tissue around the lump, as well as the lump itself, to be quite sure that the tumour has been removed fully. Because cancer often spreads to the lymph glands (nodes) in the armpit, removal of these glands is usually carried out to check whether they are affected or not. Thus a patient with a small breast tumour might have two incisions, one in the breast and one in the armpit area. In situations where the tumour is larger, extensive within the breast, or located in the centre of the breast, mastectomy (removal of the breast) is often the safer surgical approach. If this is done, the lymph glands are also removed. In the past, when a radical mastectomy was carried out, a very long diagonal scar resulted and the operation involved removal of a large amount of muscle and other tissue. The patient therefore suffered very major disfigurement and often had a serious degree of arm swelling. Today, mastectomy and removal of lymph nodes are done through a single incision and the resulting scar is usually a fine horizontal line. Muscles are not removed, significant arm swelling is most uncommon and full shoulder movements are restored. Thus the fear of many women of major mutilation, restricted shoulder movements and a painful swollen arm are remnants of another era, and patients undergoing mastectomy can at least be reassured in this respect.

Breast reconstruction

The physical and psychological effects of breast cancer and its treatment are considerable for every woman. Medical, nursing and social support, as well as the help of the family are of immense importance in recovery and rehabilitation. Patients are obviously concerned that the disease may recur either at the site of the original disease or in another part of the body. Cosmetic factors are also very relevant and restoring the form or contour of the breast may be of great importance. Thus breast reconstruction may be considered.

Breast reconstruction is rarely needed after quadrantectomy operations, although it is a consideration for patients who have had mastectomy. There are three types of breast reconstruction, or ways of restoring the breast form, after mastectomy – an external prosthesis, an internal prosthesis or implant, or a muscle-skin (myocutaneous) flap.

• *External prosthesis* – A temporary external prosthesis, in the shape and texture of the breast, is applied soon after mastectomy and before the patient goes home. A more permanent prosthesis is fitted about six to eight weeks after the operation when the scar has healed fully. The quality of external prostheses is improving rapidly. Certain forms are now available which are skin-coloured and which are applied to the chest wall with a special type of non-irritant adhesive. A suitably fitted external prosthesis can be very effective, allowing the patient to wear swimwear and evening clothes without the prosthesis being noticeable.

• *Internal prosthesis* – An internal prosthesis, made of synthetic material, is implanted behind the chest muscles to provide a breast contour. These prostheses can be implanted either at the time of mastectomy or later. The reason why these implants are not routinely inserted is that they can produce discomfort and scarring around them and do not always give a satisfactory result. Nonetheless, improvements in the technology of implantible prostheses will undoubtedly lead to their more widespread use as more suitable implant materials are developed.

• *Muscle-skin flap* – The breast contour can be restored by a surgical operation which involves the transfer of muscle and overlying skin from another part of the body to the area of the breast. The operation involves the implantation of the patient's own muscles (usually abdominal or back muscles) to build up a mound of tissue in place of the breast. This involves a major operation and is rarely done at the time of mastectomy. It often provides a most satisfactory form of breast reconstruction and does not involve the implantation of foreign material.

The choice of which type of reconstruction is most suitable depends on many technical and medical factors. For any patient, this choice should be a matter for discussion between herself and her doctor.

Radiotherapy

Radiotherapy is often an effective way of treating cancer. Some forms of cancer can be cured by radiotherapy alone. The effectiveness of radiotherapy is based on its ability to interfere with and destroy the cancer cells while protecting and preserving the normal cells of the affected area.

After breast surgery, radiotherapy is usually carried out by external beam radiation. It is generally not needed in patients who have had a mastectomy where the glands in the armpit have been removed. Radiotherapy is recommended, however, for patients who have had quadrantectomy operations. In this situation, the radiotherapy is administered to the residual breast tissue. The radiation therapy is given in small fractions and the course is spread out over several weeks in order to minimise any radiation irritation to the skin or other structures. The purpose of this kind of treatment after breast-conserving surgery is to protect the remaining breast tissue against recurrence of the disease as much as possible.

Radiation therapy is sometimes given by needle implants either into the tumour or into the breast tissue after the tumour has been removed. This treatment is carried out in special radiotherapy centres, with the patient usually attending as a day-patient.

Chemotherapy

Even after apparently curative surgery and radiotherapy, and when there is no sign of any remaining disease, the long-term outlook for patients may be improved further by chemotherapy. Chemotherapy drugs block the growth and replication of cancer cells. They also interfere with normal cells to some degree, which explains why such chemotherapy has side-effects. Even so, chemotherapy drugs are much more active and selective against cancer cells than against normal cells.

A distinction must be made between 'adjuvant' chemotherapy and chemotherapy given to patients with advanced or recurrent disease. Adjuvant chemotherapy is given to people who have had apparently curative treatment by surgery, with or without radiotherapy, in an attempt to protect the patient further by killing off any tiny cancer cells that might be lingering within the body. This form of chemotherapy usually involves the use of three drugs – Cyclophosphamide, Methotrexate and 5-Fluorouracil. The treatment course is rather prolonged and takes place over a period of about six months. In general, the drugs are administered every three weeks for nine courses. This usually involves the patient coming to hospital as a day-patient for an intravenous injection or infusion of treatment followed by a course of tablets.

There is no doubt that significant side-effects can occur from this type of treatment, including nausea, vomiting, loss of hair and interference with the body's resistance to infection. With skilled care and careful planning of treatment, however, the toxic side-effects of these drugs can be minimised. The ordeal of adjuvant chemotherapy is less frightening and distressing than was the case even ten years ago. This form of treatment is generally advised for younger women before the menopause, particularly if there is any sign of disease in the lymph glands.

Hormonal therapy

Some patients are more suitable for hormonal therapy than for chemotherapy after initial surgical treatment. Such patients fall into two categories – post-menopausal women and pre-menopausal women whose tumours have oestrogen receptors.

• *Post-menopausal women* – The hormonal therapy given to post-menopausal women is Tamoxifen. This treatment has a complex type of hormone action by interfering with the uptake of oestrogen in tissues and blocking the growth of tumours. Tamoxifen is given in tablet form and is remarkably well tolerated. It is generally prescribed for two years or for five years and confers additional protection against recurrent disease in women after the menopause.

• *Pre-menopausal women with oestrogen receptors* – Some tumours have the ability to trap oestrogens in receptors within the cells of the tumour. These receptors can be detected in the laboratory. The patients whose tumours have oestrogen receptors might be more suitable for hormonal therapy instead of, or in addition to, chemotherapy. In pre-menopausal women, the most suitable hormonal therapy involves blocking the function of the ovaries. This can obviously be done by removing the ovaries or by radiotherapy, but such treatment permanently abolishes the function of the ovaries. This means that the patient cannot have any more children and undergoes an early menopause. The most advanced way of interfering with ovarian function is by an injection that interferes with hormone production by the ovaries. This type of biochemical method of abolishing ovarian activity has the advantage of being reversible once the treatment has been discontinued.

FOLLOW-UP CARE

In spite of the best possible treatment, some patients develop a spread of the disease which becomes apparent at follow-up examination. Breast cancer can spread to other parts of the body, such as bone, lungs, liver or brain; such spread is referred to as metastases or secondaries. When breast cancer recurs in other areas of the body, it can still be treated with radiotherapy, chemotherapy and hormonal therapy, but the long-term outlook after the development of secondaries is generally poor.

It is now fully understood that follow-up nursing, medical and counselling services are required by patients who have undergone treatment for breast cancer. Medical and nursing check-ups at regular intervals have generally been found to be of physical and psychological help. Support groups can also be of great benefit. Reach to Recovery is the best known of these groups and has done an enormous amount of good in offering practical help and advice to women who have had breast cancer. It is undeniable that most patients who have had this disease suffer significant psychological upset and some may develop reactive psychiatric disturbances. It is most important that such patients are identified and helped at an early stage.

THE LONG-TERM OUTLOOK

People should no longer be fatalistic and assume that breast cancer is invariably fatal. It is not. Huge efforts in research are continuing worldwide to understand further the biology and causes of breast cancer. It is disappointing that no cure is yet in sight. However, significant advances have been made in the understanding of the disease in terms of its basic biochemistry, biological behaviour and spread. Significant advances and refinement in treatment have also been made. Public information about the issue is becoming more widespread. The medical profession is becoming more informed and more communicative about the condition.

For patients with small tumours and in whom the lymph nodes are not affected, over 90 per cent are alive and well twelve years after treatment. It is true that the outlook is not so good in patients with large tumours, particularly if the lymph nodes are affected, but the excellent results associated with top quality investigation and treatment for small tumours augurs well for the future.

Useful addresses
Reach to Recovery, Irish Cancer Society, 5 Northumberland Road, Dublin 4. Tel. (01) 6681855.

Europa Donna, Piazza Tricolore 2, 20129 Milan, Italy.
Europa Donna is a European women's movement which is active in the fight against breast cancer.

———————————

Niall O'Higgins BSc, MCh, FRCS Eng, FRCS Ed, FRCS Ire is Professor of Surgery at University College, Dublin, and a Consultant Surgeon at St Vincent's Hospital, Dublin.

COUGHS AND WHEEZES

PROFESSOR M X FITZGERALD

Coughing isn't exactly the stuff that poetry is made of, yet Shakespeare described winter with an image we can all appreciate.

When coughing drowns the parson's saw,
... and Marion's nose looks red and raw.

Professor Muiris FitzGerald is a consultant in respiratory medicine, and as such he deals mainly with the very serious lung conditions such as cystic fibrosis. But in this chapter, he looks at the more common conditions that cause coughs and wheezes.

We have all experienced coughing when we have had a cold or flu. Smokers cough when they light up the first dreaded weed in the morning. We have all coughed and spluttered when 'something went the wrong way' while eating too fast. Parents know all about cough – nothing is more calculated to drive you crazy than a child coughing all night and interrupting everybody's sleep. Teachers will tell of the frustrations of trying to teach a class of five-year-olds during the winter when the latest cold virus is doing the rounds, with the entire class creating a racket with their incessant coughing. Go to any concert hall, theatre or church and listen to the din of coughing that breaks out after a quiet piece of music, the end of the second act or when the sermon is over. So, it seems, cough is a common experience for young and old, particularly during winter. That fact alone is reassuring – most coughs are not due to any serious medical condition. They come and go, and affect all of us at one time or another, especially when we have a cold or flu.

But common experience also tells us that a cough that goes on for a long time or that is accompanied by breathlessness or phlegm streaked with blood can mean something more serious. John Wayne and Steve McQueen both developed prolonged, unusual coughs and chest discomfort, and both were found to have lung cancer. Countless Victorian novels portrayed heroes and heroines who languished away, having coughed blood into their handkerchiefs and eventually died of consumption, the disease we know as tuberculosis. So it appears that certain types of cough can herald some more serious and occasionally sinister underlying disease of the lungs. Obviously, that raises important questions – what is cough, and, more importantly, how do we separate the innocent short-lived cough of winter colds from the more worrying cough that might mean lung cancer, tuberculosis or some other serious condition of the respiratory system?

WHAT IS COUGH?

A cough is one of the most vital defence reflexes in the body because it protects the lungs from irritation, injury or damage.

First, there is a sharp intake of breath as we suck air into our lungs quickly. This is followed by an explosive movement of the chest, where we expel air with great velocity and force. At the same time, we tense and narrow the air passages in our throat, which gives rise to the strained, grunting, rasping sound of a cough. When something irritates the air passages of the lung, this triggers a protective reaction of the lung designed to expel any irritant. Thus, if a particle of food, instead of being swallowed, goes with our breath, the lung will instantly respond with a powerful cough to expel the particle. If we have a winter cold with irritation of the lining of the air passages or some sticky mucus blocking the air passages, a powerful cough will shoot the pellet of mucus up the air passage towards the throat so that it can be coughed up and the obstruction relieved.

If we did not have a powerful cough reflex, then food and liquid would get into our lungs and we would die of pneumonia. Similarly, we need a cough as a warning signal that some irritant condition is developing deep in our lungs.

There are many ways to sub-divide cough. The simplest way of categorising it would be as follows: (1) the simple, straightforward cough; (2) the persistent cough where it would be wise to consult a doctor; (3) the cough requiring immediate medical consultation.

Simple, straightforward cough

This usually occurs in winter with colds. It may be accompanied by nasal stuffiness and mucus, and minor sore throat. Other members of the family may be affected. Occasionally, mild fever may be present. The individual gradually gets better and is never really terribly sick at any time. Such simple, straightforward cough is never accompanied by major wheeze, marked breathlessness or croup and never features symptoms like coughing up blood. Common examples of this type of cough include simple winter colds, minor flu viruses, minor allergy and post-nasal drip (mucus sliding down the back of the throat from the nose, particularly at night).

The persistent cough

This is a more protracted cough with slight elements of croup or wheeze, discoloured mucus, slight breathlessness, persistent fever with general fatigue and tiredness. Common examples are more severe flu and virus infections, troublesome bronchitis, emerging asthma, early mild pneumonia, allergic conditions of the lung or a change in pattern of a smoker's usual cough.

The cough requiring immediate medical consultation

This involves any cough accompanied by any of the following – streaks of blood in the phlegm, severe breathlessness, high fever particularly when accompanied by shaking chills, severe wheeze, croup or severe malaise, a general feeling of being unwell. Examples of such more severe and serious causes of cough include pneumonia, severe obstruction of the upper respiratory passages, particularly in children, tuberculosis, lung cancer, fibrosis of the lung, clots in the lung, heart failure, and regurgitation of acid and food from the stomach into the lungs. You should consult your doctor immediately. If your doctor is not available, go to the accident and emergency department of your nearest adult or children's hospital.

THE DOCTOR'S APPROACH TO COUGH

During a clinical examination, a careful history is taken, and the chest and throat are examined. It may then be possible to come to a diagnosis relatively simply, or further investigations may be needed. These may include straightforward ones which can be done at the doctor's surgery, such as a blood test, sputum (phlegm) test or breathing test. A more complicated level of testing may be necessary, however, with referral for a chest X-ray or to a specialist.

If a cough is very unusual, complex, persistent or accompanied by danger signals, a hospital investigation may be necessary. This may include sputum analysis, more sophisticated breathing tests, or chest X-rays and scans. An internal examination of the lungs could be required. Here, a flexible telescope (called a bronchoscope) is passed down the throat into the lungs and an internal view is obtained. Various samples and scrapings of the lung may also be taken.

Treatment of cough

In most cases, this may just involve waiting until it goes away, or the prescription of simple remedies such as cough syrup may ease discomfort. Giving up cigarettes or avoiding smoky, dusty atmospheres may be important preventive measures. If a specific cause has been identified, appropriate treatment is prescribed. Examples include antibiotics for chest infections, preventive inhalers for asthma or anti-inflammatory medications (steroids) for certain types of lung inflammation. Specific medical or surgical treatments might be indicated for very complex lung disorders such as lung cancer, lung clots or lung fibrosis.

WHEEZES

Wheezes are high-pitched, squeaky, piping sounds that come from the air passages of the lungs when they are narrowed or congested. They can usually be heard when somebody with a condition like asthma takes a deep breath quickly or, more often, when they breathe out rapidly and compress their lungs, giving rise to these characteristic musical sounds. The sounds are sometimes compared to the high register of the bagpipes, an old accordion or worn-out bellows. Another sound that comes from the lung is called stridor. This is a close first cousin of wheeze but is invariably heard on taking a breath in. Stridor sounds like the initial 'hee' of a donkey's 'hee-haw'.

The sounds of wheezes and stridor are due to turbulent vibrations of air caused by the breath being forced through air passages that are markedly narrowed. Narrowing of the air passages of the lung can occur due to one or more of the following mechanisms: (1) inflammation and swelling of the lining of the air passages (bronchial tubes); (2) excessive accumulation of sticky mucus in the air passages; (3) spasm and constriction of the muscles that surround the bronchial tubes; (4)

sometimes, an obstruction by a solid particle of food that has gone the wrong way and blocked an air passage; (5) very rarely, a cancer that grows into the passageway of an air tube and blocks it partially or completely.

These are obviously the mechanical ways in which the air passages can be narrowed – but what are the common conditions that will give rise to wheeze? Doctors have a simple rule of thumb for wheeze in teenagers and adults – persistent wheeze means asthma until proved otherwise. The emphasis is on the word persistent, because it is a common experience that occasional wheezy noises and rattles can occur briefly and temporarily during a flu or cold in individuals who do not have asthma. It is the continuation or repeated recurrence of wheeze that signals asthma as the prime suspect.

CHILDREN WHO WHEEZE

Most children with asthma will have cough and wheeze. But because of the narrower air passages in children, simple colds and attacks of bronchitis can also cause wheezing in the earlier years of life. Therefore, it is sometimes difficult to be certain in young children whether wheezy colds represent simple temporary narrowing of the bronchial tubes by mucus, or whether it reflects a possible underlying asthmatic tendency. Parents of young children and their doctors sometimes have to adopt a 'wait and see' policy with wheezy colds in children.

ASTHMA

The condition known as asthma is the most common cause of wheezing in adults and children. So it is worthwhile looking at a few characteristics of wheeze which can be valuable pointers in further confirming asthma. Wheeze of asthmatic origin is frequently aggravated by the following factors:

• Exposure to household dust (hoovering, sweeping), domestic aerosols (fly killer, deodorants, perfumes, oven cleaner), soft furnishings such as pillows and duvets filled with feather or down.

• Close contact with domestic animals such as cats, dogs,

hamsters and budgies which generate hairs, dander and animal fluff.

• Passive cigarette smoking in enclosed spaces like pubs, clubs and discos, or at social functions where people smoke.

• Seasonal and weather changes – in some asthmatics, wheeze can be prominent in May and June due to grass pollen in the air or in the winter when there are a lot of fungal spores in the environment.

• Rapid changes in temperature such as going from a warm house out into the cold in the winter time.

• Exercise – most asthmatics note that they become tight and wheezy when they run quickly.

• Chest infections – wheeze often flares up when common winter cold and flu viruses are doing the rounds.

• Intense emotional stress – a small proportion of asthmatics will notice a tensing of their chest and the emergence of wheeze when they are under sustained emotional pressure such as domestic or business stress or following bereavements.

• Occupational factors such as exposure to dust, fumes, gases and vapours generated in paint and plastic manufacture, soldering operations, and in the fine chemical and pharmaceutical industries.

WHEEZING AND SUSPECTED ASTHMA

Consult your doctor who will listen carefully to your chest to confirm the audible wheeze and then go on to carry out simple breathing tests. The standard approach is to blow into an air velocity gauge called a peak flow meter which records the speed and efficiency with which you can blow out air from your lungs. If you have a wheeze due to narrowing of the air passages, you will register a lower than normal score on this machine. If your peak flow is low, that suggests obstruction of the air passages.

A diagnosis of asthma can be confirmed by a further test. Your doctor will get you to breathe several puffs of an anti-asthma spray (inhaler) which relaxes the tightened bronchial muscles.

This relaxation of the tight muscles leads to a relaxation of the spasm, an opening up of the narrowed air passages and, not surprisingly, a far better score on the peak flow meter some ten to fifteen minutes after the asthma spray. An improvement of more than 10-15 per cent in the peak flow recording virtually clinches a diagnosis of asthma and there is no need for any additional expensive and sophisticated testing. Occasionally, however, if your doctor is in doubt, arrangements may be made for a specialist consultation with a respiratory physician, a chest X-ray or any other necessary tests. But usually asthma can be readily diagnosed when your doctor takes a careful history, records the presence of wheeze and documents an improvement in your peak flow measurement after the administration of an anti-asthma medication inhaler.

TREATING ASTHMA

The general approach for treating asthma is one of regular preventive treatment at two levels.

• Avoid aggravating factors such as dusts, fumes and vapours as much as possible. Common measures include getting rid of feather pillows and duvets, covering the mattress with an oil cloth (to keep down the highly allergenic house dust mite), avoidance of strong-smelling sprays and aerosols, and elimination of smoke from smoky fires or persistent smokers.

• Regular preventive asthma medications are prescribed. These are usually in the form of simple spray inhalers which are taken every morning and night to soothe the allergic irritation of the lung and to eliminate spasm and constriction of the bronchial muscles. These preventive medications are supplemented from time to time by occasional puffs of a bronchodilator aerosol which temporarily relieves transient spasm of the lungs when quick relief is needed.

LIVING WITH ASTHMA

Asthma is a readily controlled condition with an excellent outlook, provided regular treatment is taken year round to prevent the problem. It is very much like the preventive approach to dental decay. You brush your teeth twice a day to maintain good dental health. Similarly, regular preventive anti-asthma treatment does the same job in protecting your lungs.

Supervision of treatment for asthma is usually carried out by your family doctor or, if the problem is more complicated, by a specialist respiratory physician. But you are the most important person of all to keep a close eye on your asthma. That is why most doctors will put newly-diagnosed asthma patients through a comprehensive education programme. This instructs them about the nature of their condition, the indications for medication, a contingency plan for what to do in a crisis and a regular means of monitoring their own condition. This latter factor is very important, and with the introduction of simple peak flow meters which can be obtained at a very reasonable price, asthmatics can monitor their own condition very accurately from day to day or from hour to hour. By having such an objective early warning system, the asthmatic with wheeze can accurately assess his/her condition and adjust the treatment according to a pre-arranged plan as set out by their doctor. In that way, the person with asthma is empowered and can feel a sense of control over a condition which is usually life long. Furthermore, many people with asthma find it fruitful to join an association like the Asthma Society which keeps the asthma community up-to-date on all the latest world trends in diagnosis, treatment and monitoring.

Useful Address
The Asthma Society of Ireland, 24 Anglesea Street, Dublin 2. Tel. (01) 6716551.

M X FitzGerald MD, FRCP, FRCPI, FRCPEd, FCCP is Professor of Medicine at University College, Dublin, and a Consultant Physician in Respiratory Medicine at St Vincent's Hospital, Dublin.

DEPRESSIVE ILLNESS

PROFESSOR PATRICIA CASEY

*In the past, many terms were used to describe this condition –
reactive depression, endogenous depression, neurotic
depression, psychotic depression, clinical depression. However,
because there is an overlap between all these conditions, the
medical profession has decided to abandon these terms and to
talk simply about depressive illness and manic-depressive illness.
Manic-depressive illness is characterised by major mood swings
from elation to depression and it is quite rare.*

*Patricia Casey, Professor of Psychiatry at University College,
Dublin, discusses the more common forms of depressive illness.*

THE DISTINCTION BETWEEN
UNHAPPINESS AND ILLNESS

Depression is a term that has multiple meanings, some of which differ when used in the medical as distinct from the lay context. First and foremost, depression describes a mood state that covers a range of emotions, from boredom, spiritual despair and tearfulness through to profound hopelessness. Indeed in its most severe form, there is the absence of all emotional responses so that even crying is impossible. The word 'depression' is so non-specific that when someone says they are feeling depressed, it may be no more than the understandable feelings of despondency we all feel during bad weather, when worried about a problem or after a bereavement. On the other hand, it may also be indicative of a depressive illness.

The distinction must be made between unhappiness and depressive illness so that the sufferer gets the correct help. Someone who is suffering from unhappiness does not have a medical problem and may only require counselling and support. However, someone who has a depressive illness can benefit enormously from the appropriate medical treatment.

The essential difference between the two is that unhappiness decreases as time progresses, allowing a person to adapt and cope. This also occurs if the stress is removed – a person who is in debt inherits money and is able to discharge that debt. If the mood changes persist despite the passage of time or the removal of the stress, then it is likely that a depressive illness has developed and that medical treatment is required. When the stresses are persistent, such as with long-term poverty or marital disharmony, it is impossible to decide what might happen should the situation alter. The distinction between illness and unhappiness is thus very difficult.

SYMPTOMS OF DEPRESSIVE ILLNESS

These can be divided into two major groups. The first are emotional in nature, while the second are physical. Surprisingly, the physical manifestations of depressive illness are more prominent than the emotional ones.

Physical symptoms

The most common symptoms are those of anxiety, including sweating, palpitations, chest pain, stomach discomfort, nausea, urinary frequency, dry mouth, headache and dizziness. At their most severe, these may lead the patient to believe that he/she is having a heart attack, often culminating in admission to a coronary care unit for assessment. It is common for patients to be referred to cardiologists, gastroenterologists or neurologists for investigation of suspected heart disease, peptic ulcer or some other physical disorder.

Other prominent physical symptoms include appetite loss and sleep disturbance (usually under-sleeping but occasionally sleeping to excess), accompanied by feelings of exhaustion and aches and pains. Sometimes more definite pain is prominent, especially in the back and face. The insomnia and exhaustion may lead to difficulties in carrying on with the daily routine; when time has to be taken off work, employment may be jeopardised. Not surprisingly, a patient with this range of symptoms is often diagnosed as having a viral infection.

Emotional symptoms

The most prominent feelings are those of tension and worry or depression. The patient may be suffering from a general feeling of anxiety. On the other hand, their worries may become focused on something that seems very minor to everyone else. They may blow up small details of their lives out of all proportion to their importance. Depressed mood may not be described directly, but rather as a lack of all emotion, as a sense of greyness or as a cloud over day-to-day living. Patients also describe a feeling of being out of control, sometimes leading to a terror of impending insanity. Not all depressed patients cry and indeed some are unable to, although they wish they could.

111

Irritability is common and is directed at those in immediate contact with the patient. If associated, as often happens, with a loss of sexual interest, the marital relationship can be seriously impaired. Loss of confidence is common, and fear of going out or of meeting people may occur in tandem with the physical symptoms of anxiety. A mistaken diagnosis of agoraphobia is therefore sometimes made. Increasing dependency on family members may be of such severity as to make it difficult for the partner to go to work or to leave the patient alone. Memory and concentration are also impaired and feelings of hopelessness are common. Among some patients, suicidal ideas, either fleeting or more fully developed, occur and may lead to attempts at deliberate self-harm, either with the motivation of committing suicide, but more commonly as a way of drawing attention to their plight – the typical 'cry for help'.

Patients with depressive illness describe their depression and anxiety as being worse in the morning.

PREVALENCE

Depressive illness is more common in women than men by a ratio of three to one. It can occur in any age group, even in children, but it peaks in the thirty-five to forty-four age group. In general, the later the age of onset, the more severe the illness. Studies show that it is present in between 10 and 13 per cent of the general population. It is thus the most common emotional disorder. There is no relation to social class. Only about 10 per cent of those with depressive illness are referred to psychiatrists. Most are treated successfully by their general practitioners.

CAUSES

Stressful events

Depressive illness is often, though not always, triggered by a specific event. Not surprisingly, many people look for causes; when none are found, they will evoke trivial events to explain the illness. Among the factors that provoke depressive illness are a whole range of 'loss' events, such as bereavement through divorce, separation, death, miscarriage, stillbirth or induced abortion. Not all the provoking events are negative, and even positive events such as childbirth may also be associated with depressive illness. There is no evidence to link the menopause to this illness, although folklore does make this connection. Other less obvious loss events such as moving house or leaving a job can also provoke a depressive illness.

Physical illnesses
A range of physical illnesses and medical treatments are themselves associated with depressive illness. These include painful bony conditions such as rheumatoid arthritis, thyroid gland disorders, hysterectomy, amputation, coronary artery bypass operations and steroid treatment.

Childhood experiences
There is no evidence that an unhappy childhood causes depressive illness, although it may make the individual more vulnerable to such an illness. However, childhood experiences may lead to other problems such as eating disorders, alcoholism, anxiety and phobias. Indeed many people who develop depressive illness have no such background of unhappiness and come from supportive and stable families. Sexual abuse in childhood is often followed by depressive illness in adult life, but most of those with depressive illness have no history of sexual abuse.

Personality
As with childhood experiences, there is no specific association between personality and depressive illness, although those who are dependent or obsessional may be more vulnerable in the face of negative life events. It is true to say, however, that most of those who develop this illness are well adjusted and stable in their personalities.

Neurochemical
Regardless of whether there is a definite stress factor or whether

there is a background vulnerability, it is believed that all depressive illness is the result of a change in brain chemistry. The chemicals particularly involved are nor-adrenalin and serotonin. This is why antidepressant drugs are prescribed even when the illness has been triggered by some external stress or event.

TREATMENT

Most people with depressive illness can be treated by their GPs without referral to psychiatrists. At present, only about 10 per cent of patients are referred. However, when the symptoms of depression are present, it is essential to seek help, since untreated depressive illness can lead to deterioration in relationships with one's spouse or partner and children, work problems, and suicide in a minority of cases. The attitude of 'I want to cope with it myself' is mistaken and leads to prolonged suffering.

Chemical

In the first instance, this involves breaking down the symptom barrier so that the patient's view of the world can become positive. He/she can then begin do deal with the trigger, if indeed there has been a definite one. To achieve this symptom reduction, antidepressants are required. These are non-addictive and can bring about symptomatic recovery within a few weeks of commencement. All antidepressants take a minimum of two weeks for their effect to begin. Thereafter, improvement is gradual rather than dramatic, with patients describing a gradual 'lifting of the cloud'. At times it may be necessary to try several antidepressants before one is found to be successful. There is no known reason for this, although the level of antidepressant achieved in the brain may be responsible. The common antidepressants are Tricyclics (Amitriptyline, Dothiepin and Cloimipramine), Tetracyclics (Mianserin and Maprotoline), Monoamine oxidase inhibitors (Tranylcypromine, Phenelzine) and specific serotonin re-uptake inhibitors (Fluoxetine, Sertraline). Other antidepressants include Trazodone and

Lithium. Antidepressants also have uses in addition to their antidepressant role, as in the control of bulimia and manic-depression. Side-effects include blurred vision, dizziness, dry mouth, constipation, drowsiness and difficulty in passing urine.

In the first instance, treatment will need to be continued for at least six months following improvement in symptoms if a rapid relapse is not to occur. In the elderly and in those who suffer recurrent episodes, antidepressants may need to be continued for life to prevent disabling recurrence. During treatment, the patient can continue to work and function, provided the severity of depression does not preclude this.

Electro-convulsive treatment (ECT) is rarely used nowadays. Its main and almost exclusive use is for severe depressive illness (depressive psychosis) in which there is a serious suicide risk and when the patient has lost touch with reality so that he/she may believe that she/he is possessed by the devil, for example.

Psychotherapy
In addition to drug treatment, the patient may need to deal with events that may have provoked the illness, such as bereavement or sexual abuse. There is a mistaken view among many patients that such psychotherapy cannot take place while taking pharmacological treatments. This is untrue, and the only limiting factor in treatment is the ability of the patient to engage in psychotherapy – an area most likely to be compromised by the severity of the patient's depression due to an inability to be detached and to view the issues realistically. It is therefore essential to break down the symptom barrier with antidepressants before proceeding with psychotherapy. It is obvious that where there is no triggering factor involved, no in-depth psychotherapy is required, other than to reinforce the patient's sense of self-worth during treatment and to encourage an early return to the day-to-day activities that have been compromised by the illness.

A recently developed form of psychotherapy is cognitive therapy. This focuses on the patient's here-and-now feelings and attempts to redirect the patient's negative thoughts. Unfortunately, despite early claims of success in prevention of relapse, these have not been universally shown. It is also very labour intensive, requiring up to thirty hours of therapy before symptoms resolve.

OUTCOME

If untreated, depressive illness can and does lead to untold suffering. Marital relationships are strained, work is compromised and the inability to form attachments to one's children can have a negative impact on them. The use of alcohol to relieve symptoms has its own attendant problems which will compound those that already exist. Symptoms persist indefinitely, although interestingly, the most severe forms of depressive illness, for example those warranting admission to hospital, can often disappear spontaneously if left untreated. There is a mortality from suicide among those whose depressive illness is untreated; the figure of 15 per cent is often quoted, although this gives the wrong impression, since it refers to the most severe form of the illness (depressive psychosis). The persistence of anxiety, of low self-esteem and of inertia will, if not treated, lead to an indefinite 'suffering in silence'.

If treated, most patients with depressive illness make a complete recovery and roughly 70 per cent have only one episode. Every person who believes he/she may be suffering from depression should seek help, either from the family doctor or from a psychiatrist of his/her choosing.

PREVENTION

There is no evidence that any psychiatric disorders, with the exception of alcohol and drug abuse, can be prevented. In spite of this, it is important to minimise the effects of stresses by dealing with them. The ability to talk through problems with friends, spouses, partners or spiritual advisers is important, since this will assist in the ventilation of feelings and ultimately in achieving objectivity about the stress. The expression of emotions such as anger, sadness or guilt is commonly avoided, but may greatly reduce the emotional complications of bereavement. The shared experience and support from self-help groups, be it following a miscarriage, an abortion or the death of a loved one, can have a potentially preventive effect, although many find they are unsuited to the group experience and therefore should not be coerced in any way into this approach.

MYTHS

• Counselling/psychotherapy is the preferred treatment for depressive illness.

• Psychotherapy to explore the cause cannot be used while on medication.

• Antidepressants are addictive.

• Depressive illness can only be treated if the 'underlying cause' is found.

Patricia Casey FRCPsych, MD is Professor of Psychiatry at University College, Dublin, and is a Consultant Psychiatrist in the Mater Hospital, Dublin.

GROWING OLD

PROFESSOR DAVIS COAKLEY

People are now living longer than at any time in history. Although health problems can occur at any age, some are more common once we reach our sixties and seventies.

There is a growing interest in the whole area of medicine for the elderly, with the result that many conditions that were once considered an inevitable part of the ageing process are now being properly diagnosed and successfully treated.

Professor Davis Coakley is Director of the Mercer's Institute for Research on Ageing at St James's Hospital in Dublin. He explains why there has never been a better time for growing old.

GROWING OLD

The fact that most people can now look forward to a long and healthy life is one of the great achievements of modern man. During this century, there have been dramatic increases in the average life expectancy. Throughout history, of course, there has been a small group of 'biologically elite' who lived into old age, some even surviving into advanced old age. However, even in comparatively recent years, the change has been dramatic. The number of centenarians in the UK has increased from around 250 in 1950 to about 4000 today.

Two Irish women famed for their long lives were the sixteenth-century Countess of Desmond and the Honourable Katherine Plunket who died earlier this century. The Countess of Desmond, who lived in the castle of Inchiquin near Youghal in Co. Cork, is said to have lived to be 140. According to one of her contemporaries:

> She might have lived longer had she not mette with a kind of violent death, where she must need climb a nutt tree to gather nutts, soe falling down she hurt her thighe, which brought a fever, and that brought death.

The Honourable Katherine Plunket of Ballymascanlan House, Co. Louth, was born in 1820. She was an enthusiastic gardener, and in September 1931, when in her 111th year, she won a prize at the Dundalk show for her fruit and vegetable exhibit. She died a year later when she was almost 112 years old.

AVERAGE LIFE EXPECTANCY

Although there are now over 400,000 people aged over sixty-five in the Republic of Ireland, forming more than 11 per cent of the total population, Ireland still has the lowest life expectancy in the EC. The sixty-year-old European female can expect to live another 22.1 years on average, compared with only twenty years for the Irish female. The mean for the sixty-year-old European male is nearly eighteen years, while it is only sixteen years for the Irish male. From these figures, it is clear that, on average, women live four years longer than men, and that people in

Ireland die, on average, two years earlier than the average European.

The main causes of death in Ireland are heart disease, cancer, lung disease and stroke. The fact that there is now more emphasis on a healthier lifestyle, as well as an increased awareness of good health care in later years, should improve the life expectancy of the average Irish person. A seventy-five-year-old woman can now expect to live for another ten years, a fact that emphasises the importance of good health care in old age. Ten years is a long time in a person's life, so everything possible should be done to ensure that the years are of high quality. While this is desirable for humanitarian reasons, it also makes good economic sense in this increasingly mercenary age.

A UNIQUE POPULATION PROFILE

People are living longer now because of improved environmental factors. Better housing, clean water, improved sewerage systems, healthier diets – all of these have played a part. In the past, old age was the privilege of the few. Now, it is regarded as the birth-right of all. We need a fundamental rethink on the whole subject of growing old. We must accept that most people expect to live long lives. It should therefore be our aim to make the quality of a person's last twenty years as good as the previous years.

SOME MISCONCEPTIONS

It is a common error to view the elderly as a single homogeneous group. Yet they are as different as any other age group in society. There are the usual distinctions associated with current or previous employment, social status and education. Although problems with health certainly are more common for those over seventy-five, even in advanced old age, the majority of people still live at home.

There is a general assumption that health and physical ability decline remorselessly with advancing years. This is simply not the case. One study carried out by Duke University in the US followed a group of elderly people over several years. They found that half of those who returned regularly for assessment suffered no decline in physical ability during periods ranging from three to thirteen years.

Sexuality in older years has been a taboo subject for many years, yet research has shown that many older people still enjoy enriching and fulfilling sexual relationships. Couples who share an active sexual relationship in their younger years usually continue this relationship as they grow older.

Ageing is part of the natural cycle that begins at conception and ends with death. It is therefore important to distinguish between chronological age and biological age. Two people aged seventy might have been born on the same day, but they may have aged at different rates, making one biologically much younger than the other. Even in the same person, organs can age at different rates. For example, the heart of one seventy-year-old person may compare favourably with that of a sixty-year-old, even though other parts of the body such as the skin may be more like that of the typical seventy-year-old.

Changes associated with ageing should not be confused with those caused by disease. Changes associated with ageing do not cause significant disability on their own. Complaints should never be dismissed with glib comments such as, 'What can you expect at your age?' If such a question is posed, the appropriate answer should be, 'Good health care!' People should be aware of the importance of distinguishing between the changes associated with normal ageing and those associated with illness. The treatment of illness in old age, as at any age, can bring about remarkable improvements in a person's quality of life.

OLD AGE AND MODERN MEDICINE

Despite the fact that older people can live healthy and active lives, there is still an unacceptably high level of illness associated with age. Conditions such as Parkinson's disease, Alzheimer's disease, arthritis and stroke all impair the quality of life for a small but significant percentage of older people. This fact presents modern medicine with one of its greatest challenges. At

122

the beginning of this century, serious illness and disability were common in childhood and accepted as part of life. The concentrated efforts of pioneering paediatricians and medical scientists changed this situation so that serious illness in childhood is now unusual. The illnesses of old age are now being tackled by an increasing number of physicians and medical research institutes who specialise in the medical problems of the elderly. Consequently, many more people will be able to grow old without major disabilities.

Experts who make gloomy predictions about ageing often assume that, over the next twenty years, people will age in the same way that people did in the last twenty years. This is a fundamental error. People who are growing older today are far healthier than older people of a similar age twenty or thirty years ago.

AGEING SKIN

Contrary to popular opinion, ageing itself does not produce many changes in the skin. Thin skin, pigment changes and wrinkles are mainly caused by exposure to the sun. Ultra violet light is also responsible for the hard or keratotic patches seen on the faces of some older people. It also causes skin cancers, including malignant melanoma. Some older people can develop very thin skin, especially on the backs of the hands and the forearms. This is harmless and is the result of poor elasticity in the skin tissues. These changes can also lead to easy bruising which is slow to resolve. Itchiness can be due to excessively dry skin, although there can be other causes. If it persists, a doctor should be consulted.

VISION

Eyesight should be checked regularly as it can be affected by a variety of ageing and disease processes. A rapid build-up of fluid pressure within the eye can cause severe pain, blurred vision and vomiting. This condition needs urgent treatment.

More commonly, pressure can build up gradually and lead to

an insidious loss of eyesight. People are often unaware that this condition, known as glaucoma, can have a silent and painless onset. A considerable amount of vision can be lost before it is detected.

There are several causes of sudden visual disturbance in older people. An acute change is always a medical emergency. It should be reported to a doctor immediately, as urgent action is often required if the vision is to be saved.

Most people have heard of cataract formation which is caused by an opacification of the lens. However, it is still surprising that many people allow their vision to go almost completely before they seek help. Modern technology has revolutionised the treatment of cataracts.

Some older men and women develop a condition known as macular degeneration which damages the retina and leads to marked visual problems. High magnification lenses can be helpful in dealing with this problem.

HEARING PROBLEMS

It has been estimated that over half of older people develop hearing problems. There is an age-related decline in the ability to hear higher frequencies, and this makes it particularly difficult to hear consonants. As consonants convey much of the sense of speech, high frequency loss can greatly impair an individual's ability to follow a conversation.

Age changes in hearing begin in middle age. They often become apparent when a person experiences an increasing difficulty in following conversations, especially when there is any background noise. Those who have significant high frequency hearing loss can be helped with a hearing aid. Modern aids are quite sophisticated in design and function. They amplify certain frequencies and have noise-suppression units that make it easier to follow speech in a noisy environment.

Impacted wax is a common and treatable cause of hearing loss. The amount of moisture within the ear canal declines with age so that wax secreted by the skin glands tends to become dry and hard. Removal of this wax can 'cure' the resulting deafness.

Whatever the cause of a hearing loss, it is important that it should be investigated and treated early. If deafness is ignored, the person who is affected can become socially isolated and depressed.

MUSCLE AND BONE

The density of bone tends to decline in both sexes from the fourth decade. Excessive thinning of the bone structure, known as osteoporosis, can lead to fractures of the limb bones or of the small vertebral bones of the spine. Loss of bone density can affect women, particularly after the menopause. This may be stopped by the use of hormone replacement therapy (HRT).

Among the other causes of osteoporosis are lack of exercise and an inadequate diet. An adequate intake of calcium and vitamin D is essential for healthy bones. Vitamin D is found in fish oils and margarine and, to a lesser extent, in eggs. Milk fortified with vitamin D is now available commercially. The body can also make its own vitamin D if the skin is exposed to sunlight. If vitamin D is lacking, normal strong bone is replaced by poor-quality soft bone, a condition known as osteomalacia. Apart from bone changes, osteomalacia can also lead to muscle weakness. The condition causes bone pain, weakness, difficulty in walking and recurrent fractures.

There are some age-related changes in the joints. However, the decline in joint function most commonly found in later life is due to osteoarthritis. In this condition, the cartilage is damaged and the joints become painful and swollen.

There are several methods of treating osteoarthritis, including physiotherapy and medication. Joint replacement can also revolutionise the quality of life for many with this severe disease. (There is further information in the chapter, 'Arthritis and Rheumatism'.)

BLOOD PRESSURE

Blood pressure tends to rise with age, and doctors accept higher levels as 'normal' for older people. The decision about whether to treat high blood pressure in old age is based on factors such as the level of the pressure, any evidence of damage to organs such as the heart and brain, and whether the person will be able to tolerate the treatment involved. Blood pressure should be checked periodically as part of a routine medical assessment, as significant and untreated high blood pressure can lead to conditions such as stroke.

INTELLIGENCE AND MEMORY

Contrary to popular opinion, there is little evidence to suggest that intelligence declines with age. There may be some loss in the speed and flexibility of response, but this is often compensated for by the better judgement that comes with experience. In one study, for example, older bus drivers had poorer results than younger ones when tested in an artificial situation using computer simulators. However, the older drivers performed better than their younger colleagues when asked to drive a bus in hazardous test conditions. A study of musicians in one of America's great symphony orchestras found that older musicians were highly valued for their excellence and experience, and many did not retire until they were well over seventy.

It is common for older people to complain about some degree of forgetfulness. This is usually harmless and rarely develops into a significant problem. Some people, however, do suffer from much more marked forgetfulness. When memory loss begins to cause concern and to interfere with the quality of one's life, it should be reported to a doctor.

There are many illnesses that can cause memory impairment; some of these, such as vitamin B_{12} deficiency, can be treated. In the past, older people who became confused were described as being senile and little was done for them. But as a result of considerable research over the last two decades, we now know that so-called 'senile' people are suffering from one of a number of conditions that affect the brain. The most common of these is Alzheimer's disease. Although great advances have been made in the methods used to diagnose this condition, the underlying cause has not yet been found. Medical scientists are optimistic about progress in this area and relatively effective remedies may appear on the market within the next decade.

Multi-infarct dementia is another common cause of chronic confusion in the elderly. In this condition, small areas of the brain are damaged over a period of time by a series of minor strokes. The person is usually unaware of these events but eventually, intellectual ability becomes impaired as the damaged area increases. It is more common in older patients with high blood pressure. There is some evidence to suggest that effective control of blood pressure, combined with small-dose aspirin therapy, may slow the progress of this condition.

Any significant memory loss is not a part of normal ageing. It is due to an illness which should be investigated like all other illnesses.

EXERCISE

Research indicates that some of the decline in physical ability that occurs in old age may be attributed to decreased levels of physical activity and exercise. This emphasises the importance of maintaining fitness throughout adult life. Studies have shown that healthy seventy-year-olds can be trained to a level of physical performance which is comparable to that of forty-year-olds. The level of exercise should be graduated to suit the individual. It would be unwise for older people to embark upon vigorous new exercise programmes without first consulting their doctor. The potential for improving the physical performances of elderly people is greater than had been suspected and does not depend on having been a fitness enthusiast in earlier years.

EARLY IDENTIFICATION OF PROBLEMS

One important message for older people and their families is that many of the problems traditionally ascribed to old age are in fact due to various disease processes. Falls, incontinence or increased immobility are often caused by a treatable illness and should never be dismissed as being due solely to old age. Treatment has a much greater chance of success if a doctor is consulted early.

It is often suggested that older people do not need the facilities of high-technology hospitals for the investigation and treatment of their illnesses, and that they merely block access to these facilities for more deserving younger patients. This is not true. Older people have benefited greatly from advances in medical technology. They can now be investigated and treated more accurately and more safely than ever before. Advances in surgical and anaesthetic techniques have also made surgery much safer for older people.

Consulting a doctor as soon as possible is important when significant problems develop. However, it is important to sound a word of caution. As they grow older, most people develop a number of minor problems, so the temptation to demand a pill for each complaint is often great. Over time, such an approach can lead to serious disability because of over-medication. Good medical practitioners are aware of this and do not rush for the prescription pad on each consultation.

OLDER PEOPLE IN SOCIETY

Older people have much to offer society, and it is important that they are encouraged to play active roles rather than passive ones. There are many ways in which this might be done. In the last decade, there has been a growing demand for more flexible retirement schemes which would move away from the idea of mandatory retirement at sixty-five. Such schemes would allow some individuals to retire earlier and others to remain at work for longer, depending on personal choice and the circumstances of the posts involved. These schemes could be introduced without blocking employment opportunities for younger people.

Anyone who is about to retire should take advantage of the pre-retirement courses that are now available. These programmes concentrate on issues such as finance, health and leisure, and, as at all ages, it is sensible to plan ahead.

There are many ways in which older people can continue to

contribute to society in a voluntary capacity. Ireland has a particularly strong tradition of voluntary community developments, and retired people can contribute their skills in a wide variety of ways. Able and healthy older people can therefore do much to help their less fortunate contemporaries who have been disabled due to illness.

Older people also have more time to develop their intellectual and artistic skills. There is now an increasing emphasis on older adult education with courses ranging from the very academic to the extremely practical.

The best guarantee of a healthy and fulfilled old age is to follow the ancient classical concept of being fit in mind and body. There are many examples in literature and the arts of people who have remained creative and active even into advanced old age.

Professor Davis Coakley MD, FRCPI is Consultant Physician in the Department of Medicine for the Elderly, and is Director of the Mercer's Institute for Research on Ageing at St James's Hospital, Dublin. He is currently President of the Irish Gerontological Society and Dean of the Faculty of Health Sciences at Trinity College, Dublin.

HEART DISEASE

PROFESSOR IAN GRAHAM

About 15,000 people in Ireland die each year from diseases of the heart and arteries, especially heart attacks and strokes. This accounts for about half of all deaths, and makes them the biggest single cause of death, greater than all cancers, infections and accidents combined. Other forms of heart disease include disease of the heart valves, and congenital heart diseases such as a hole in the heart.

In this chapter, cardiologist Professor Ian Graham writes mainly about heart attack and angina, the two major manifestations of coronary disease. He describes how we can prevent heart disease and help ourselves to stay healthy. Because there is much confusion about the medical terms that are used in this area, he also includes a glossary at the end . . .

THE SYMPTOMS AND SIGNS OF HEART DISEASE

Apart from the fact that it is the major cause of death in Ireland, there is another reason why heart disease, particularly coronary heart disease, is an important health issue. The hardening of the coronary arteries (atherosclerosis), which causes heart disease, develops over many years. Many of the causes of atherosclerosis come from the way we live. Therefore the answer to coronary heart disease lies with the whole community rather than with the medical profession alone. Countries such as the United States, Canada, Australia and Finland which have traditionally had high death rates from heart disease have adopted lifestyle changes such as cutting down on smoking which have helped to reduce their death rates from heart attack.

The most common symptom of heart disease is chest pain, although most people who attend heart clinics complaining of such pain turn out to have normal hearts. Chest pain can be caused by problems in the food pipe, in the lungs, even from the abdomen. Many people also experience stabbing left-side chest pains, especially when tired or stressed, and these are seldom due to heart disease.

Angina is characterised by a particular type of chest pain which tends to occur when the heart speeds up in response to emotion or exertion. The pain is usually in the middle of the chest (rarely to the left), and is tight or squeezing in character. It may spread to the neck or jaw, to the arms, and less commonly to the back or the abdomen. The pain is usually strong enough to make the person stop exercising, at which time the feeling generally subsides quickly. Angina pain that comes on more and more easily is sometimes called unstable angina and may require admission to hospital.

The pain of a heart attack is similar to that of angina, but often comes when the person is at rest. It is usually more severe and lasts longer, often for hours. There may be sweating and fear with the pain. Although such pain does not always mean a heart attack, it is usually wise to seek medical help promptly – most people who die from a heart attack do so within the first few hours, often while they are still wondering whether to seek help or not.

When a patient with a heart attack is examined, everything may appear normal, although the heart rate is often fast. Other findings depend on the seriousness of the attack. An electro-cardiogram (ECG) reading often shows a characteristic pattern, but not always. In doubtful cases, doctors usually recommend admission to hospital, since ECG and blood test changes may take some time to occur.

Although most chest pains do not come from the heart, a bad pain such as the one described, especially in a middle-aged man, requires immediate medical help. Doctors are just as relieved as their patients when the pain is an innocent one. The rule is: better safe than sorry.

THE CAUSES OF CORONARY
HEART DISEASE

While some illnesses such as infections have a single cause, it has taken a long time to work out the many specific reasons for coronary heart disease. The major risk factors, which appear to actually cause heart attacks, are a high fat diet which results in increased blood fat (cholesterol) level, cigarette smoking and high blood pressure. Lack of exercise, stress, family history, diabetes and many other factors may increase the risk of heart attack, but do not have as strong an effect as the big three risk factors.

Heart attacks are more common in the middle aged and the elderly. This is so because older people have been exposed to risk factors for longer. Heart attacks are also rare in women up to the time of menopause, although death rates increase from then on.

FOOD – TOO MUCH OF
A GOOD THING?

Many people are confused about the relationship between diet and heart disease. This is partly because scientific evidence on

133

the subject is rather complicated. In addition, inaccurate information has been published by vested interests and self-styled experts possessing only a limited knowledge of the subject.

The facts, however, are relatively straightforward. In countries such as Ireland, people eat more saturated (hard) fats of animal and dairy origin than they need and have high blood cholesterol levels as a result and thus higher death rates from heart attacks. Populations whose diets are low in fat (such as the Japanese) or contain more vegetable fats (such as Mediterranean countries) have lower death rates from heart attacks.

Because many other factors relate to heart attacks, it is reasonable to question the association with a high-fat diet. However, evidence from studies of heart patients, animal experiments, post-mortem studies and studies of diet in many countries indicate that a high-fat diet does indeed cause heart attacks.

Hard (saturated) fat in the Irish diet comes from meat, dairy products and confectionery. Both meat and dairy products are nutritious foods. The problem is that many of us eat more of these foods than our bodies need.

The Irish Heart Foundation has examined the relationship between diet and heart disease in detail in its *Irish Heart Foundation Nutrition Policy*, a report that summarises the recommendations of various institutions.

Dietary recommendations for fat intake

Expert panel	Population recommendations % energy as	
	Total fat (%)	Saturated fat (%)
World Health Organisation (WHO)	30	10
US Consensus Conference	30	10
European Atherosclerosis Society	30	10
British Cardiac Society	35	15
Irish Heart Foundation	35	12 (short term)
	30	10 (long term)

Such recommendations are pretty well meaningless unless translated into actual food-stuffs. For this reason, the Irish Heart Foundation Nutrition Policy has also prepared a table outlining food choices that will help to lower blood cholesterol levels and hence the risk of heart attack.

	ADVISABLE	IN MODERATION	NOT ADVISED
CEREAL FOOD	Wholemeal flour, oatmeal, wholemeal bread, wholegrain cereals, porridge oats, crispbreads, wholegrain rice and pasta cereals	White flour, white bread, sugarcoated breakfast cereals, white rice, pasta	Fancy breads, eg croissants, savoury cheese biscuits, cream crackers
FRUIT AND VEGETABLES	All fresh and frozen vegetables – peas, broadbeans, sweetcorn. Dried beans and lentils are very high in fibre. Baked potato – eat skins. Fresh and dried fruit.	Avocado pears, olives	Potato crisps, chips
NUTS	Walnuts	Almonds, Brazil nuts, chestnuts, hazelnuts, peanuts	Coconuts

FISH	All white fish, oily fish eg herrings, tuna	Shellfish occasionally	Fish roe
MEAT (LEAN)	Chicken, turkey, veal, rabbit, game	Ham, beef, pork, lamb, bacon, lean mince, liver and kidney occasionally	Visible fat on meat (including crackling), sausages, pâté, duck, goose, streaky bacon, meat pies, meat pastes
EGGS AND DAIRY FOODS	Skimmed milk, low fat milk, skimmed milk cheese eg cottage and curd cheese, Egg white	Edam cheese, low fat Cheddar, Camembert, Parmesan, 3 egg yolks per week only	Whole milk, cream, hard cheese, Stilton, cream cheese. Excess egg yolks
FATS	All fats should be limited	Margarine labelled 'high in polyunsaturates', corn oil, sunflower oil, soya oil	Butter, dripping, suet, lard, margarine not 'high in polyunsaturates', cooking/ vegetable oil of unknown origin
MADE-UP DISHES	Skimmed milk puddings, low fat puddings eg jelly, sorbet, skimmed	Pastry, puddings, cakes and biscuits made with suitable margarine or oil and	Tinned or whole milk puddings, dairy ice cream, pastry, puddings,

	milk sauces, cakes and biscuits made with suitable margarine or oil and wholemeal flour.	white flour, ice cream	cakes, biscuits and sauces made with whole milk, eggs or unsuitable fat or oil, all proprietary puddings and sauces, mayonnaise
SWEETS, PRESERVES AND SPREADS	Bovril Oxo Marmite	Meat and fish pastes, boiled sweets, fruit pastilles, peppermints etc. Jam, marmalade, honey, sugar	Peanut butter, chocolate, toffees, fudge, butterscotch, lemon curd, mincemeat
DRINKS	Tea, coffee, mineral water, unsweetened fruit juices, clear soups, home-made soups eg vegetable, lentil	Packet soups, alcohol	Cream soup

NOTES

1. Foods ADVISABLE are generally low in fat or high in fibre. These should be used regularly as part of your diet.

2. Foods IN MODERATION contain polyunsaturated fats or smaller quantities of saturated fats. As your diet should be low in fat, these foods are allowed in moderation. For example, a) red meat not more than 3 times a week; b) medium fat cheeses and meat and fish pastes once a week; and c) homemade cakes, biscuits and pastries made with suitable polyunsaturated margarine or oil, twice a week.

3. Foods NOT ADVISED contain large proportions of saturated fats and therefore should be avoided wherever possible.

4. For overweight people, avoid foods high in sugar and limit use of suitable fats and oils.

In simple terms, a healthy diet should include the widest possible variety of foods. In the Irish context, an increased use of vegetables, fruits, cereals and fish will help to moderate the consumption of high-fat foods. In addition, convenience foods, snacks and confectionery should be avoided since they tend to be high in saturated fats.

People with a high blood cholesterol level are three times as likely to have a heart attack. The risk is greatly increased if they smoke or have high blood pressure. These facts point to the need for a holistic approach to health – diet is important, but it is only one of several risk factors.

While the relationship between fat intake and heart disease is definite, there is still more to be learned about diet. Recent research suggests than certain vitamins may help to protect against heart attacks in several ways. Vitamins C and E may make cholesterol less damaging to the arteries. Folic acid and vitamin B_{12} may lower the levels of a substance called homocysteine which may also be associated with heart attack. A wide and varied diet will ensure the adequate intake of these substances. In the future, nutritional guidelines may concentrate more on foods that include these vitamins.

SMOKING

Cigarette smoking, like a high-fat diet and the resultant high blood cholesterol, increases the risk of heart attack about three-fold (see the chapter on 'Smoking'). Smoking also increases the risk of stroke, bronchitis, emphysema, lung cancer and a number of other cancers. Smoking is also unpleasant for other people, and non-smokers may suffer a slightly increased risk of disease as a result of others' smoke.

It is doubtful whether anyone in Ireland does not know that cigarette smoking is bad for health. Indeed the habit is gradually dying out here. Twenty years ago, 40 per cent of adults smoked. The figure is now down to one quarter of adults, and it is now not acceptable to smoke in public places or at work. Nevertheless, it should be realised that smoking is highly addictive and that smokers need our help and support if they are to abandon the habit.

BLOOD PRESSURE

Raised blood pressure also increases the risk of heart attack and stroke. It greatly increases the risks associated with high blood cholesterol and cigarette smoking. In most people, high blood pressure does not cause any symptoms, so the only way to know whether or not your blood pressure is raised is to have it measured by a doctor. Today, there is great interest in finding ways of controlling high blood pressure without the use of drugs. Reducing weight, avoiding the contraceptive pill and cutting down on salt consumption can all help. Once again, this points to the value of fresh, unprocessed foods, since most convenience and processed foods contain large amounts of salt.

LACK OF EXERCISE

People who are active, who take vigorous exercise four or five times a week, have a lower risk of heart attack than inactive people. Some of this protection may come from the exercise, but much of it comes because such people are often interested in what they eat, are less likely to be overweight and are unlikely to smoke. Exercise is also a good way of reducing stress.

STRESS

Many people who experience a heart attack believe that it was brought on by stress, although the evidence that stress causes heart attack is weaker than is generally supposed. There is some evidence that worry, frustration and anger may damage health, although everyone experiences these feelings to some extent. Stress is certainly a less important risk factor than high blood cholesterol, cigarette smoking and high blood pressure.

FAMILY HISTORY

Heart attacks do seem to occur more in some families than in others. While the tendency to heart attack or to suffer from risk factors such as high cholesterol may be inherited, in many cases the explanation is more simple. Lifestyle habits such as cigarette smoking and a high-fat diet tend to run in families. This makes knowledge of a healthy lifestyle all the more important to people with a strong family history of heart attack. In some people, the problem is definitely inherited; for example, some cases of very high cholesterol levels. In such people, drug treatment for high cholesterol may be needed as well as dietary advice.

OTHER RISK FACTORS

Certain other conditions may increase the risk of heart attack. These include an underactive thyroid gland (hypothyroidism) and diabetes. Both of these conditions can be controlled with medical treatment.

Many of those factors that cause heart attacks can be controlled by our own actions without recourse to medical help. We can decide upon a healthier diet and make the decision not to smoke. High blood pressure can only be detected if it is checked regularly, but this only takes a few seconds. Active people have lower risk levels, and exercise also reduces stress. A few minutes' thought about what one eats or making time for an enjoyable form of exercise will not guarantee freedom from heart disease, but they will certainly improve one's chances for a long, happy and healthy life.

INVESTIGATING HEART DISEASE

The most important point of investigation begins with a person's description of their symptoms, be it chest pain, breathlessness or some other symptom. By listening carefully, the doctor will often know quite quickly whether or not heart disease is likely. Further medical investigation may be necessary, either for reassurance or as a means of confirming the presence of heart disease. This will include a blood pressure check, a test of the blood fats (particularly cholesterol), a chest X-ray and an ECG. In doubtful cases, an exercise ECG may help. A coronary angiogram is sometimes required for absolute certainty. It is always needed if a patient has definite angina that has not responded to medical treatment and that may require angioplasty or coronary artery bypass graft surgery. With modern techniques, a coronary angiogram is an easy test, although the complicated equipment may look rather frightening. The test carries a very small risk, which should always be explained fully before it is undertaken.

TREATMENT AND RECOVERY

Many cases of angina resolve with straightforward advice about diet, moderate exercise, stopping smoking, controlling high blood pressure and simple medication. In more severe cases, narrowed coronary arteries can be dealt with either by balloon angioplasty or by coronary artery bypass graft surgery. Although not completely free of risk, these procedures are now very safe; 97 per cent of patients undergoing heart surgery will recover.

It is important to note that the occurrence of angina, even heart attack, is a beginning, not an end – most people make a full recovery and return to full and normal lives. Many hospitals now run rehabilitation programmes. The word 'rehabilitation' means 'return to normal life'. These programmes aim to help patients by providing information about diet, exercise, drugs and so forth. If you have been diagnosed as being at risk of heart attack, of having angina, or if you have already had a heart attack, it is quite reasonable for you to ask your doctor for the fullest possible advice about your long-term future so that you can remain well and healthy.

COMMUNITY ACTION

The realisation that we can all take positive action to reduce our risk of heart disease has led to the development of a number of community initiatives throughout Ireland. The first of these was the Kilkenny Health Project. Aided by the Irish Heart Foundation and the Health Promotion Unit of the Department of Health, it aims to provide lifestyle advice for people in Co. Kilkenny. Arising from this, the Irish Heart Foundation has responded by developing Happy Heart programmes in many communities.

These include school programmes, health-at-work programmes, information about diet, help with stopping smoking and other aspects of risk evaluation.

MEDICAL JARGON TRANSLATED

cardiac: of the heart.

artery: a blood vessel (tube) that carries blood from the heart around the body.

coronary artery: the artery feeding the blood into the heart muscle to allow it to work properly. The two coronary arteries, left and right, arise from the main artery of the body (the aorta) just above the heart. They travel downwards over the surface of the heart muscle. The left coronary artery has two main branches, the left anterior descending and the circumflex.

vein: blood vessel (tube) carrying blood to the heart.

atherosclerosis: hardening and narrowing of the arteries. Any artery in the body may be affected. If the coronary arteries are affected, angina or heart attack may occur. If the arteries to the brain are affected, stroke may occur.

angina: a chest pain that occurs when the heart muscle is not getting enough blood, particularly when it speeds up in response to exercise or emotion. The usual cause is narrowing (atherosclerosis) of the coronary arteries.

heart attack: damage to the heart muscle caused by complete blockage of a coronary artery. Usually causes angina-type pain, but is more severe and longer lasting. Other names for heart attack are coronary thrombosis and coronary attack.

stroke: damage to the brain caused by blockage of an artery bringing blood to the brain. Usually causes weakness (paralysis) of the side of the body, often with difficulty in speaking properly.

cholesterol: a fatty substance in the blood. Essential for life, but too much causes atherosclerosis. Another less-well-known blood fat is triglyceride. Collectively, blood fats are called lipids.

lipid: the medical term for fat. Hard fats in the diet (mostly from animal or dairy sources) are called saturated fats. Soft fats (mostly from vegetable sources) are called mono- or poly-unsaturated fats. An excess of hard fats in the diet increases blood cholesterol as well as the risk of heart attack.

electro-cardiogram (ECG): a recording in which the electrical activity generated as the heart beats is recorded on paper. The odd-looking squiggles that result may show a characteristic pattern in angina or heart attack.

exercise electro-cardiogram: an electro-cardiogram performed before, during and after exercise, usually on a moving belt (treadmill). Electro-cardiogram changes indicating angina may only show up on exercise.

coronary angiogram: a special X-ray that shows up the coronary arteries and any narrowing that may be present. A small tube is placed in the artery at the top of the leg or at the elbow, and then passed through the main arteries to the heart. It is wiggled into the origin of a coronary artery and a liquid is injected which shows up the coronary arteries on X-ray. It is used to diagnose coronary artery disease when there is doubt. Also used to outline blockages that may need angioplasty or coronary artery bypass surgery.

coronary angioplasty: similar to an angiogram, except that a tiny balloon is passed through an area of narrowing in a coronary artery and inflated to stretch the narrowed piece. May avoid the need for coronary artery bypass surgery, although this may still be necessary when two or three arteries are narrowed.

coronary artery bypass graft surgery (CABG): an operation in which pieces of leg vein (or an artery called the internal mammary which runs inside the chest wall) are used to bypass narrowed segments in coronary arteries. One end of the graft is stitched to the main artery of the body (the aorta) just above the heart. The other end is stitched into a coronary artery beyond an area of narrowing or blockage to bring more blood to the heart muscle. Very effective in relieving angina.

Useful address
The Irish Heart Foundation/The Family Heart Association, 4 Clyde Road, Dublin 4. Tel. (01) 6685001.
The Irish Heart Foundation has produced a number of leaflets on heart disease. They offer a counselling service for heart patients and their families. Their book, *Heart Attack and Lifestyle*, is available by post.

The Family Heart Association is a support group for people with an inherited cholesterol problem.

Ian Graham FRCPI, FCCP is a Consultant Cardiologist at the Charlemont Clinic, St Vincent's Hospital, the Meath Hospital and the Adelaide Hospital, Dublin. He is Professor of Cardiology at Trinity College, Dublin.

INDIGESTION AND ULCERS

PROFESSOR COLM O'MORÁIN/ DR JOAN GILVARRY

The treatment for ulcers has been revolutionised over recent years. The traditional diet of milk puddings and boiled fish is a thing of the past. The first step in modern treatment was the development of drugs that healed the ulcer. The second step was the discovery of a bacteria (Helicobacter pylori) in the gut which was causing the ulcer in the first place. The research directed at killing this bacteria was pioneered in Ireland by Professor Colm O'Moráin at Trinity College, Dublin.

Here, Professor O'Moráin and Dr Joan Gilvarry deal with ulcers and their treatment, as well as the very common complaint of indigestion . . .

INDIGESTION

Doctors describe patients as having dyspepsia when the patients themselves say they have indigestion. Dyspepsia is from the Greek words 'dis', meaning 'bad', and 'peptein', to digest. The word 'indigestion' is derived from Latin, but the two words otherwise have the same construction and the same meaning.

Dyspepsia can be defined as any recurrent pain or discomfort in the upper alimentary (digestive) tract which may be intermittent or continuous in nature and which has been present for one month or more. The upper alimentary tract consists of the oesophagus, the stomach and the duodenum.

Indigestion is a common and frequent reason for consultations with GPs and for hospital referrals. Indigestion is usually self-limiting and responds to simple treatment with antacids such as Rennies, Aludrox, Maalox or Bisodol. On occasions, however, it can be persistent, and the cause might require detailed investigation before diagnosis is made and treatment commenced. The causes of prolonged indigestion are reflux oesophagitis, gastric (stomach) ulcer and duodenal ulcer.

REFLUX OESOPHAGITIS – HEARTBURN

The gastric juices in the stomach which break down food contain acid. This is kept in the stomach by a muscular valve. Heartburn occurs when the acid secretion in the stomach is regurgitated back into the oesophagus (the food canal running from the mouth to the stomach). It is caused by acid being in the wrong place, or by the valve being defective, not by the production of an excess amount of acid.

Acid in the wrong place can cause inflammation of the oesophagus and thus pain, the main symptom of which is heartburn. It is estimated that over 150,000 Irish adults suffer from heartburn daily. Heartburn is best described as a burning pain in the chest which rises towards the throat. The pain is usually mild, but it may be so severe that patients suspect that they are having a heart attack. Heartburn is aggravated by smoking, alcohol, hot foods or beverages, fatty or spicy foods, being overweight, bending, stooping, wearing tight clothing, and pregnancy.

Investigation

• The patient's history

The progression of symptoms, together with a physical examination, will help the doctor decide which patient needs further assessment. Those who have severe symptoms for a prolonged period and who are taking large quantities of white medicines such as Maalox and other antacids should be investigated. Patients who complain of a sensation of difficulty in swallowing (dysphagia) should always be assessed further.

• Endoscopy

This is sometimes called gastroscopy. It is a test that allows the doctor to look directly into the lining of the oesophagus (gullet), the stomach and around the bend of the small intestine (duodenum). The endoscope is a long, flexible tube, thinner than your little finger, with a bright light at the end.

To do the test, the tip of the endoscope is passed through the mouth and into the stomach. Looking down the tube, the doctor gets a clear view of the lining of the stomach and can check whether or not any disease is present. Sometimes the doctor takes a biopsy – a sample of the lining of the stomach for analysis in the laboratory. A small piece of tissue is removed painlessly through the endoscope using a tiny forceps.

To allow a clear view, the stomach must be empty. The patient is therefore asked to fast for at least six hours prior to the test. It may take up to ten minutes for the doctor to examine all the relevant areas. In most cases, the doctor can give the results to the patient straight after the test. However, if a sample (biopsy) has been taken for examination, the results may take several days.

• Barium swallow and meal

This simple test, which will demonstrate most abnormalities, is carried out in the X-ray department. The patient fasts for the test and is asked to drink white liquid (barium) which shows up clearly on the X-ray. The test usually takes between fifteen and thirty minutes.

Treatment

Heartburn can be helped by a number of lifestyle changes. These include stopping smoking, losing weight and changing eating habits. Patients should avoid excess alcohol, coffee, chocolate, and foods that are spicy, fried or fatty. It is also necessary to eat little, often and slowly, making sure to chew food properly. More vegetables, fruits and high-fibre foods are recommended. Eating late at night, especially just before going to bed, should be avoided. Bending and stooping should be done correctly by bending the knees and keeping the back straight. It will also help if sufferers avoid tight clothing, especially around the waist.

When sleeping, the head of the bed should be raised slightly. Sometimes, sleeping on the left side may help.

During pregnancy, women should eat sensibly. Weight gain should be kept within the recommended guidelines.

It is surprising how often these simple remedies can help cure the problem of heartburn. Where they fail, however, drug treatment is often necessary.

• Antacids

These include white medicine, sodium bicarbonate, calcium bicarbonate, magnesium and aluminium salts. Antacids have been used for years to treat indigestion. They help to 'mop up' some of the acid in the stomach. While these agents alleviate the symptoms, they are of little or no value in the more severe cases which must be referred to hospital. Nevertheless, antacids remain the backbone of the treatment in minor cases of reflux.

• H2 receptor antagonists

Ranitidine, Cimetidine, Famotidine and Nizatidine are in this group. These tablets decrease the amount of acid in the stomach, but only about 60 per cent of patients respond satisfactorily.

• Omeprazole

This is the first of a new class of drugs that reduce acid and is the most useful one available today for the management of reflux. It leads to improvement in the majority of patients who do not respond to treatment with H2 antagonists. It offers an attractive alternative to those who might otherwise need surgery.

• Prokinetic agents

These are drugs that alter the contractions of the upper gastrointestinal tract. Metoclopramide, Domperidone and Cisapride are all beneficial. Their main value is that they increase gastric emptying and improve the efficiency of the valve between the oesophagus and stomach.

Complications

Oesophageal narrowing (stricture) is a complication of prolonged oesophageal reflux, even though the symptoms may have been very mild. The patient will complain of difficulty in swallowing, initially with solids and then with liquids. This narrowing can be dilated at the time of endoscopy. Because of the success of medical treatment in the management of reflux oesophagitis, few patients are now referred for surgery. When surgery is performed, it can now be done using a laparoscope (keyhole surgery), which has two major advantages: the patient is not left with a large abdominal scar, and the hospital stay after surgery is reduced by about 50 per cent.

Uncomplicated gastro-oesophageal reflux in young patients may be managed by the self-help measures already described. Those who fail to respond should be investigated, as medical treatment is usually successful. Surgery may be performed where medical management has failed to alleviate symptoms or complications.

ULCERS

The word 'ulcer' means 'open sore'. A peptic ulcer is an open sore in the lining of the wall of the alimentary tract, be it the oesophagus, stomach or duodenum. These ulcers are tiny, about 15mm in length, similar in size to mouth ulcers. Although duodenal and gastric ulcers are usually grouped as one, there are distinct differences in their history, treatment and follow-up procedures.

In the western world, there is a steady increase in the prevalence of ulcer disease with age, peaking for duodenal ulcers in men aged between forty-five and fifty-five. Duodenal ulcers affect some 10 per cent of the population. There has been a steady decline in the ratio of males to females with ulcers, and they now affect women almost as much as men. There is usually a family history of ulcers. The peak incidence of gastric ulcers is in the sixth decade, and about ten years later than for duodenal ulcers. Gastric ulcers are slightly more common in males.

Smoking is a major factor in ulcer diseases. The use of pain-killing drugs (non-steroidal anti-inflammatory drugs) has also been shown to cause ulcers. Stress, alcohol and caffeine consumption have been incriminated but none are strongly proven. Emotions can have a profound influence on the alimentary tract, but there is little evidence to support the concept of an 'ulcer personality'. Nevertheless, it is possible that stress may be an exacerbating factor in an individual who is prone to developing an ulcer.

Helicobacter pylori is a bacteria that lives in the lining of the stomach. First described in 1983, it is now known that this infection is a major cause of ulcers. Over 90 per cent of patients with duodenal ulcers and 70 per cent of those with gastric ulcers have been found to have this bacteria in the lining of the stomach. Treatment of ulcers should therefore be aimed at killing this bacteria.

Pain is the most frequent symptom. This is usually central and high up in the abdomen. It is experienced less often at the sides of the abdomen or belly button (umbilicus). Only in rare cases do ulcers give rise to pain in the lower part of the abdomen. The pain is usually described as gnawing, knife-like, a deep ache, tearing, or severe hunger. A duodenal ulcer pain occurs classically at night or during fasting; it may either be helped or made worse by food. Pain is related to food in 50 per cent of patients with duodenal ulcers. Gastric ulcer pain, on the other hand, appears to be aggravated by the intake of food. It is impossible, however, to diagnose the problem from the description of the pain alone. The intensity of the pain bears no relation to the size of the ulcer, and increased severity does not indicate pending bleeding or bursting (perforation). In duodenal ulcer patients, 15 per cent have bleeding (vomiting up blood or passing black bowel motions which represent stale blood from the upper gastrointestinal tract, a condition known as melaena). Only 1 per cent of patients will have perforation.

Vomiting may occur during severe bouts of pain. It may sometimes be induced, as it affords relief. During exacerbations, mild weight loss is frequently observed, but the weight is rapidly regained when the symptoms improve.

On examination of the patient, the only sign is tenderness of the abdomen, although this may or may not be present.

Diagnosis
Endoscopy is the most accurate method of diagnosis. A barium meal may also be recommended. While doing the endoscopy, samples (biopsies) may be taken from the stomach and examined under a microscope to see if there is any evidence of inflammation. A breath test is also used which can demonstrate the presence of *Helicobacter pylori*.

Treatment
The aims of ulcer treatment are the relief of symptoms, the healing of the ulcer, and the prevention of relapse and serious complications such as bleeding. Patients should avoid foods that cause irritation, such as peppers, garlic, chilli and coffee. They should eat regular meals and avoid late-night snacks. Smoking should be stopped and alcohol should be avoided, especially on an empty stomach. Pain-killing drugs should also be avoided unless they are absolutely essential.

Medication
Antacids which are available over the counter will help the symptoms by 'mopping up' the acid, but they have no role in healing the ulcer. Up until recently, H2 antagonists were the most frequently used form of treatment. They were shown to heal ulcers in between 80 and 90 per cent of cases, but had no effect on the organism. Because of this, it was likely that the ulcer would return once the treatment was discontinued. Treatment aimed at both healing the ulcer and killing the bacteria is now the

mainstay. This usually involves taking a four-week course of bismuth while also taking two different antibiotics during the first week of treatment. This has been shown to heal the ulcer and to kill the bacteria in over 90 per cent of cases. Recent evidence has shown that once the bacteria has gone, it is extremely unlikely that the ulcer will return. The endoscopy should be repeated four weeks after finishing treatment to check that the ulcer has healed and that the organism is dead.

Surgery
Because of improvements in medical treatment, it is now rare for patients with ulcers to be referred for surgery. The main reasons for surgery are bleeding or perforation. Failure of medical treatment is now very rarely an indication.

Indigestion is a common complaint. In the UK, about seven million people (17 per cent of the population) take indigestion medication at least once a week. Some 76 per cent of these have never consulted a doctor before doing so.

Patients who suffer from indigestion for a prolonged period should consult a doctor. Those who fail to respond to conventional treatment should be further investigated. Medical treatment (ie drugs) is usually successful. Surgery may be performed but it is now rarely necessary because of improvements in medical treatment.

Colm O'Moráin MD, MSc, FRCPI is Professor of Gastroenterology at Trinity College, Dublin, and is a Consultant Gastroenterologist in the Charlemont Clinic and the Meath Hospital, Dublin. **Dr Joan Gilvarry MB, MRCPI** is a lecturer in medicine at the Meath Hospital, Dublin.

INFERTILITY

Professor Robert Harrison and his team at
RCSI and the Rotunda Hospital

Well-meaning queries such as 'Anything stirring?' or 'Any news?' can be very upsetting for a couple who are trying unsuccessfully to start a family. Going for fertility tests and treatment is a long and expensive process which can itself add to their anxieties. Reproduction is one of our basic instincts, and it is understandable that those who don't achieve this can feel cheated.

With modern advances in treatment, the problem of infertility can now be solved in many cases. But just because something can be done doesn't mean it has to be done. It is important to remember that many couples enjoy happy, fulfilled lives without children.

This chapter, which covers investigation and modern treatment for infertility, has been written by Professor Robert Harrison and the Human Assisted Reproduction Team of the Royal College of Surgeons in Ireland and the Rotunda Hospital . . .

The number of couples who have difficulty in conceiving is unknown, but it has been estimated that at least 10 per cent of those having regular unprotected intercourse fail to conceive within twelve months. In Ireland, this would work out at over two thousand couples per year. Some of these will eventually conceive with or without help, but the rest will remain childless or have fewer children than they would like.

HOW IS A BABY CREATED?

Conception depends on a man and woman coming together and making love (intercourse). At ejaculation, his seed (sperm) is released into her vagina near the neck of the womb (cervix). It journeys through the uterus and fallopian tubes to meet her egg (ovum) which is released at ovulation. If fertilisation takes place when the sperm and egg (gametes) meet, they unite to form a zygote. This starts to divide, first into two cells, then four, then eight and so on, a process that continues during the passage back down the fallopian tube towards the uterus. Usually, by the 64-cell stage (morula), the inside of the uterus has been reached. The blastocyst, as it now known, attaches itself to the wall of the uterus. The embryo then develops. At about six to eight weeks, it is called the foetus which, at the end of approximately 280 days of life in the uterus, becomes the newborn baby. If after trying many times to make this happen and there is still no pregnancy, the couple may possibly be infertile.

WHO MAY BE INFERTILE?

Anyone can be infertile, even those who already have children. Nobody who has difficulty in conceiving should ever feel ashamed or disgraced. While it is the male's sperm that determines the sex of the child, a baby is made equally by a man and a woman. Therefore the cause of failure to conceive could be his, hers, or both. In some cases, no cause can be found (unexplained infertility).

Up to one in five infertile couples can be labelled as having unexplained infertility. Many of these will eventually conceive

154

by themselves. It may just take a longer time than for others. In some, there really will be a problem, but the present tests available may not be good enough to find out what that is.

HOW CAN YOU TELL IF YOU ARE INFERTILE?

Previous illnesses may cause a person to suspect infertility even before trying to conceive. A number of diseases and treatment regimes may cause difficulty in conception. If worried, you should consult a doctor, as should patients who have problems with intercourse or women who have scanty or no periods (menses).

However, it is more often found that the man and woman usually have no such complaints and feel quite normal. If regular unprotected intercourse during the fertile time is taking place, and if pregnancy has not occurred within a few months (twelve if a woman is under thirty-five, six months if she is over thirty-five years of age), there may then be a fertility problem.

WHAT CAN BE DONE ABOUT INFERTILITY?

Where the fear of childlessness is present and the couple wish to pursue the matter, the first and most important step is to arrange a consultation with their family doctor. By advising him/her in advance about what they wish to discuss, sufficient time can then be set aside. An infertility consultation is not something that should be hurried.

The doctor will first establish that the couple really are infertile – that they understand how to conceive and that they are not having problems with intercourse. Before referring them to a hospital clinic, the doctor may wish to perform some basic investigations. These will usually consist of examining semen and organising some tests on ovulation. The potentially infertile couple, however, should not take it as disinterest or mismanagement if they are immediately referred to a hospital clinic, usually a gynaecological clinic. A GP may decide to do this particularly if there could be a significant problem, if access to laboratories is limited, or if the couple is older.

All gynaecologists have training in reproductive problems but few units have the time or opportunity to set up the specialised service that can take infertility matters right through to the end of the road. So the couple may be referred on to an infertility clinic. Most of these operate on more or less the same lines. Going from clinic to clinic and from doctor to doctor in an endless search for what might be impossible is more likely to lead to sadness than success.

WHAT TO EXPECT FROM
THE CLINIC

No one can guarantee that all couples will end up with a baby. Indeed only about 30 per cent will be that lucky. Sometimes, it is not possible to find the cause of infertility. However, by considering the two partners together as well as separately, and by carrying out tests and examinations, the underlying reason (or reasons) for the infertility can be explained in at least 80 per cent of cases. This helps the couple to come to terms with their problem. Once the problem is understood, therapy can be started and the bonus of a pregnancy may come along.

TESTS FOR THE MAN

Sperm production and release

Investigation will usually begin with the man because these tests are simpler.

The man releases his sperm into the woman's vagina by having intercourse and ejaculating. If this does not happen, or if he does not have sufficient 'good quality' spermatozoa, the man may be infertile.

The male is tested (semen analysis or male function test) by counting the number and quality of sperm in a sample produced by masturbation into a sterile container. If the result of the first test proves to be abnormal (count below twenty million, poor motility or shape), and if the abnormality is confirmed by repeat examinations on other samples, more in-depth investigations will be needed, including blood tests for hormone levels. The man may then be referred to an andrologist (a male infertility expert, usually a urologist in Ireland).

TESTS FOR THE WOMAN

The cervix

The sperm placed in the vagina at intercourse aim to swim up to the entrance of the womb (cervix). If this does not happen, the sperm will die in the vagina. If enough sperm do not enter the vagina, or if the cervical mucus is not of good quality around the time of ovulation, sufficient numbers are unlikely to reach the ovum. This can also happen if sperm antibodies are present which cause sperm either to stick together or die. Fertilisation then is unlikely to take place.

Deposition and transport in the cervical region can be tested by microscopically examining a sample of cervical mucus taken from the woman some hours after intercourse (the post-coital test). This is similar to having a smear test. The idea is to see whether there are enough live sperm (between one and twenty) still surviving in the mucus. For this test, the couple will be required to make love 'to order'; this can be traumatic, particularly for men. When the test is negative (confirmed by repeat), more specialised investigations need to be carried out. These may include further tests for sperm antibodies and observing what happens when sperm and mucus meet for the first time (an invasion test).

Uterus and tubes

During each menstrual cycle, an egg is released from one of the ovaries. It is then sucked up into the fallopian tube and passes down to the uterus. There are a number of reasons why the ovum pick-up and the subsequent process through to implantation may not happen. The uterus may be a peculiar shape, or its lining may be diseased. The fallopian tubes could be blocked or held down (adhesions).

This whole area is best investigated through a laparoscope – a telescope which is inserted at or near the navel area under general anaesthesia. Laparoscopy is the only way of definitively diagnosing endometriosis, a common and significant problem for many infertile women in which fragments like the lining of the womb are found on or in other tissues in the pelvic cavity. In some situations, laparoscopy may be preceded or followed by a utero-tubal X-ray (hysterosalpingogram). Dilation and curettage (D and C) may be carried out and samples of the uterine lining may be taken (endometrial biopsy). Another type of telescope, a hysteroscope, may be inserted through the cervix to look at the inside of the uterus.

The ovaries

The events of the menstrual cycle (including ovulation, when the egg is released) can be looked at in a number of ways. Knowing the starting date of each period during the time the woman attends the clinic is a must. Regular periods do not guarantee normal ovulation. Ovulation is likely to take place fourteen days prior to the start of menstruation each month. If periods are regular, estimates of the likely fertile time can be made. Noting and examining cervical mucus discharge can further pinpoint the ovulation date. During the ovulatory fertile phase, the mucus is thinnest and most plentiful (the wet days). This is when it is most suitable for receiving and transporting sperm.

Taking and making a note of her temperature every morning will allow the woman to construct charts. These can also provide clues as to the time when ovulation may be taking place. It happens when the temperature is at its lowest.

Ultrasound scans of the ovary can now be used to monitor egg development in the ovary. Biochemical kits are also now available to detect hormonal secretions associated with ovulation. These may be purchased over the counter at pharmacies and used by couples to test for the 'fertile time' using the woman's urine or, possibly in the future, saliva.

However, such continuous attempts to monitor ovulation may

prove upsetting. Couples may become obsessed with the 'right time' for intercourse instead of simply making love. There is no evidence to suggest that having intercourse on an exact day increases the chance of conceiving, providing intercourse normally takes place around the time of ovulation.

The information gained from these tests is limited and inexact, and to use any such methods beyond two or three months can be soul destroying and stressful. Long-term investigative charting is not often recommended today.

At present, the most scientific and accurate way of looking at the events associated with the menstrual cycle and ovulation is through blood tests that examine the relevant hormones produced by the woman. As well as hormone tests, the woman may be asked to undergo examination of the endometrium (the lining of the womb) by D and C or to have a biopsy, a piece of ovary taken during laparoscopy for further examination. Such tests may also be helpful in those rare cases in which infertility is not due to failure to conceive but is due instead to early miscarriage.

TREATMENT

Intercourse problems

When physical causes such as disease or its treatment, congenital abnormalities of the relevant organs or hormone problems have been ruled out, psycho-sexual counselling may be recommended (see the chapter entitled 'Sexual Difficulties'. This is highly successful, particularly in the female with vaginismus (involuntary tightening of the vagina which prevents penile penetration). If the problem is that semen can be produced by masturbation but ejaculation into the vagina does not take place at intercourse, then artificial insemination with the partner's sperm (known as artificial insemination by husband, or AIH) can be used to achieve a pregnancy.

The male – semen abnormalities

There is often little that can be done when there are semen abnormalities, especially if they are severe or if no sperm at all is produced. Even when therapy is possible, it takes a long time to see if treatment has worked or not, as it takes three months to produce new spermatozoa. Statistics reveal that only 10-15 per cent of men with a treatable seminal problem succeed in making their partners pregnant.

A varicose vein on the testicle (varicocele) is commonly associated with problems of the sperm. An operation to tie off the vein may restore fertility. In relatively rare cases, hormone imbalances can be corrected. However, general measures such as having intercourse during the fertile period, maintaining a good lifestyle without smoking or drinking to excess, and wearing loose underwear and trousers appear to be just as successful as expensive drugs. Few of these drugs, if any, have been shown to give better results than placebos. In addition, the testes are designed to work at a degree or two below body temperature. If they are continually pressed up against the body by tight clothing, they won't function properly.

When the problem is severe or untreatable, or if therapy has not helped, couples may choose to bypass the problem by using donor semen. Artificial insemination by donor (known as AID) is available in at least two reputable centres in the Republic of Ireland.

At present, *in vitro* fertilisation (IVF) is not a cure for male infertility. If the man's semen is of poor quality, the results from IVF or artificial insemination are extremely poor. However, new technology is at present under development which could allow fertilisation of the oocyte by a single sperm.

In dealing with the infertile male, it is important to realise that, no matter what the semen quality is, this male is just as much a man as any other.

The male/female – the cervix
When the cervical mucus is deficient (dysmucorrohoea), oestrogen therapy may improve both quality and quantity. However, where sperm antibodies are found, this therapy is not very successful. In this situation the male can be given drugs

(steroids) but a more frequently used alternative is to try to remove the antibodies attached to the sperm by washing techniques. The resultant sample may then be placed directly into the woman's uterus, or it may be used for an attempt at *in vitro* fertilisation (IVF). The pregnancy rate from this treatment is also poor.

The female – uterus and tubes

An abnormally shaped uterus, due to either a congenital defect or the presence of fibroids (benign growths), will usually give rise to habitual miscarriage rather than total failure to conceive. Operations to restore the normal shape of the uterus may be successful but they cannot be applied in all situations. Hormonal treatment may cause the fibroids to shrink or disappear. This same therapy can be used over a number of months to treat endometriosis as an alternative to operations.

When the fallopian tubes are either blocked or unable to pick up the ovum because of adhesions, an operation may repair the damage. However, there is likely to be an enhanced risk of a pregnancy outside the uterus (ectopic pregnancy) which is potentially a life-threatening situation. When pregnancy does not occur within two years, where tubal damage is extreme, or indeed where the tubes have been removed, the opportunity to pass on to IVF should be considered.

The female – ovulation

When ovulation appears to be a problem, a number of different ovulation induction agents (fertility drugs) are available. The aim of these is to ensure that at least one ovum is produced and released in the cycles under treatment. A variety of hormones may be prescribed to treat hormonal abnormalities. When sex hormone injections are used, there is a high risk of multiple births. When properly chosen, and in the absence of any other problem, the woman who is put on fertility drugs can have a 60-

70 per cent chance of conception. The vast majority of these conceptions occur within the first six months of treatment.

NEW TECHNOLOGIES

While there may be a good deal of art, there is very little science about the act of sexual intercourse. Artificially depositing sperm into the vagina can, in many cases, be performed by the couple themselves in the privacy of their own home and at the appropriate time. This can lower the tension associated with such procedures. The sperm may come from the partner or from a donor.

When semen quality is low, it must be treated chemically and inserted directly into the uterus. This may cause problems for the woman, but new techniques are overcoming this and maximising the quality of the sperm injected.

TEST-TUBE BABIES

In vitro fertilisation (IVF) involves surgically removing an egg from the ovary and fertilising it outside the body with sperm from either the partner or a donor. The fertilised egg is then placed in the woman's uterus through the vagina. *In vitro* literally means 'in glass', and refers to the dish that is used in the process of fertilisation. This is where the term 'test-tube baby' comes from.

In vitro fertilisation was initially devised to overcome problems with the fallopian tubes. IVF and associated techniques such as GIFT (gamete intrafallopian transfer) and ZIFT (zygote intrafallopian transfer) can be effective in other fertility problems.

Because of the high-profile attention that these techniques have received from the media, invariably reporting successes rather than the more numerous failures, it can prove difficult to persuade couples that IVF is not the cure for all fertility problems. Couples should realise that only between 10 and 15 per cent of them will take babies home from the assisted reproduction unit. This puts the prognosis from the new technologies into their proper context. There is usually considerable personal financial outlay and everyone involved finds *in vitro* fertilisation extremely demanding.

All these factors should be weighed up. Before embarking on any fertility treatment or investigation, clients should understand exactly what they are getting themselves into. For many couples, however, new technology such as IVF affords the opportunity to 'close the book'. Following such treatment, a couple feels that they have tried everything possible to have children. This can give great comfort.

Robert F Harrison MA, MD, FRCS, FRCOG, FRCP is Professor and Head of the Royal College of Surgeons in Ireland Academic Department of Obstetrics and Gynaecology and Director of the Human Assisted Reproduction Unit (HARI), Rotunda Hospital, Dublin.

MEN'S PROBLEMS

MR T E D McDERMOTT

Sometimes it seems that every magazine you pick up and every radio programme you hear is full of non-stop talk about 'women's problems'. Although they are rarely mentioned, men also have problems 'down below'.

With males as well as females, there is a considerable overlap between the reproductive system and the urinary system (the water works). A urologist is the specialist who deals with urinary problems in both men and women, as well as with problems affecting the male reproductive organs.

Urologist T E D McDermott outlines the most common male problems. These are prostatism (which includes benign enlargement of the prostate as well as cancer of the prostate), impotence and testicular cancer.

PROSTATISM

The prostate is a walnut-sized gland lying below the male bladder whose only known function is to secrete some of the fluids in semen. Enlargement of the prostate generally affects men over the age of fifty. Younger men are affected occasionally, but this is rather unusual. The incidence of prostate problems increases with age, peaking in the mid sixties. It is extremely difficult to assess the numbers of men affected by this disease. However, it is recognised statistically that over 10 per cent of the population in the British Isles and over 30 per cent of the population in the United States have had medical intervention for their symptoms.

Prostate symptoms vary dramatically. They include:

• Frequency in urinating (passing urine more often).

• Poor stream of urine (the flow or power of the stream is significantly less than the normal). In some instances the stream is so wet that it dribbles on the trousers.

• Hesitancy (where there is significant delay prior to passing urine). This can occur particularly in a public place where the patient realises that other people are coming in and out and he is still waiting to start his flow.

• Incomplete emptying (despite having been to the toilet there is still the feeling that urine is left in the bladder).

• Post-micturition dribbling (the man notices a small drip in his trousers on walking away from the toilet).

• Dysuria (patients experience pain or burning on passing urine. Occasionally there may be blood in the urine.)

Prostate disease has been recognised for many years. The famous song about Frère Jacques refers to a travelling French surgeon who used to go around the fairgrounds of Europe dealing with bladder problems. Surgery for prostate disease was introduced in the mid 1800s. However, it was not until the early 1930s that surgery was regularly carried out to treat this very upsetting condition.

TREATING PROSTATE DISEASE

The treatment of prostate disease has a number of aims. It both improves the urinary flow and decreases the need for frequent urination. It also helps to avoid episodes of urinary retention (where the patient is unable to pass urine at all and is in some distress).

Tablet therapy

Tablet therapy consists of two drugs which are used to shrink different components in the prostate. These tablets have a limited success. Satisfaction rates vary between 25 to 30 per cent of patients put on this therapy. It often takes between six and twelve months before the full benefits are achieved. Patients are required to stay on tablet therapy to maintain their benefits. Side-effects for a small number of patients may include depression, dizziness, impotence and occasional skin rashes. The effects of these drugs on the sperm are as yet unclear, so they should not be used when procreation is being considered.

Prostate machines

Prostate machines heat or cool the prostate in order to kill the disease tissue. The technique has been used widely, but the results were not always satisfactory. Newer techniques using ultrasound seem initially to be more exciting, with significantly more potential. Trials using these machines are still in progress.

Balloon treatment

One further form of treatment consists of crushing the prostate using a very high-pressure balloon inserted through the penis. This technique is not widely practised. Its main limitation is that the benefits may last for only a year and may need repeating. Its main advantage is that it has no effect on erection. In some cases, however, ejaculation can be affected.

Coil or stent treatment

This is like a wire-link fence introduced into the penis and the prostate under local anaesthetic to hold the prostate open. It is generally restricted to patients who are not fit for surgery.

Various alternatives to the wire mesh have been considered, including plastic tubes. In some cases, temporary relief is achieved using these treatments, allowing alternatives to be considered if the situation improves.

Surgery

There are two methods of surgery for prostatism. In open surgery, an incision is made in the abdomen and the prostate is enucleated (removed whole). Closed surgery, which is more common, is called transurethral prostatectomy. This technique removes the prostate by scraping it out through the penis using a special electrically-powered instrument. Transurethral surgery, first described in the 1930s, is still used in most hospitals and is considered the safest technique in most situations. Ninety per cent of patients get a satisfactory result. Other treatments have yet to come up to its level of satisfaction. There are a number of advantages of this treatment over open surgery. There is a shorter stay in hospital. There is less blood loss and no scar. The procedure is also significantly shorter.

Laser treatment is now being used in some centres as an alternative, but results to date are no better than those from standard surgery.

All types of surgery can affect erection and in most cases do affect ejaculation. It is estimated that between 4 and 10 per cent of patients have problems with erection after transurethral surgery where there were none before. Ejaculation is affected by most forms of surgery. The emission goes backwards into the bladder instead of coming frontwards. However, most patients get an improved orgasm or sensation of ejaculation following transurethral surgery.

PROSTATE CANCER

Cancer of the prostate is one of the most common cancers in men. Nearly 9 per cent of deaths due to cancer are caused by prostate disease. In 50-60 per cent of cases in the EC, the cancer is not discovered until it is already an established disease and has spread to other organs. Most of these patients have a life expectancy of up to thirty-six months. Patients who have localised disease and are treated by X-ray treatment or radical surgery have an 85 per cent chance of survival after five years.

Prostate cancer is found in two ways. The patient may have the type of symptoms associated with prostatism, or they may have no symptoms at all, and the abnormality is only found on a screening exam or during prostate surgery. When cancer of the prostate is suspected, screenings include digital examination (the physician feels the prostate through the rectum), ultrasound examination, biopsy, X-rays of bones, and bone scans (nuclear imaging).

Treatment of prostate cancer

There are various treatment alternatives for prostate cancer. The condition is kept under observation through regular check-ups. Surgery, radiotherapy or hormone treatment are also possibilities.

Surgery is the most common treatment for patients under the age of seventy. If the cancer is caught in time, surgery seems to give the best chance of cure. Complications of surgery may include incontinence, impotence or infertility.

Incontinence occurs in significantly less than 20 per cent of patients. It can be controlled by the addition of an artificial sphincter if it is a long-term problem. Impotence is common in over 50 per cent of patients, but can also be treated. All patients who have this surgery will be infertile afterwards, and this condition is not correctable.

Screening

At present the nature of prostate cancer is not well understood. In many cases, despite cancer being diagnosed by biopsy, the tumour does not progress over the following years. There are, however, patients who have a progressive tumour — a tumour that will spread, for instance, into bone and cause problems.

Much discussion is going on regarding screening programmes for prostate cancer. The transatlantic view is that all males over the age of forty should have annual screens, including digital rectal exams to identify early disease and remove it. Recent research from Europe, however, suggests that such screening programmes may be of little value and result in many patients undergoing complicated surgery unnecessarily.

There is some evidence that men who have had vasectomies are at risk of developing prostate cancer in later years. Although the results of this research are not yet conclusive, it is advisable that men who have had vasectomies should be screened annually once they reach the age of fifty.

IMPOTENCE

About 50 per cent of patients with impotence are considered to have a psychological cause for their problem. (This is discussed in the chapter entitled 'Sexual Difficulties'.) Half are deemed to have a physical cause for their problem, such as reduced blood flow in, increased blood flow out or decreased nerve function. This group of patients can be helped by surgery.

Drug therapy has also been used to improve blood flow into the penis. Therapy used in America includes the drug Yohimbine. The results vary dramatically. The drug has not been considered to be of sufficient benefit to warrant its import into Ireland.

The main types of treatment used in Ireland include self-injection, vacuum devices, elastic band treatment and surgical implants.

Self-injection

The major drug used for self-injection at present is Papaverine Hydrochloride, with or without a combination of Phentolamine. These drugs are available in Ireland at a reasonable price. They are injected directly into the penis in preordained doses which must be rigidly adhered to. Satisfactory erections occur in 70-80 per cent of patients. An alternative drug therapy used elsewhere is Prostaglandins. This is not available in Ireland in dosages that would allow its regular use. At present the drug is available in high doses but it is too costly for use on a regular basis.

All drug therapy has the potential complication of priapism

(continued painful erections lasting for over four hours). If this occurs with any drug therapy, the patient must go to the nearest hospital for immediate treatment.

Vacuum therapy and elastic band treatment

These devices have an established track record. Recent innovations have included the addition of pump mechanisms to achieve an easier action. In essence, a rigid condom is applied over the penis and the air around the penis is sucked away. In doing this, the blood is drawn into the penile area and engorgement or erection is achieved. To maintain an erection, an elastic band is placed at the base of the penis. This form of erection can be maintained for around thirty minutes. Satisfaction is achieved in about 70-80 per cent of patients.

Elastic band treatments can also be used with men whose erections cannot be maintained. Simple application of these bands over the penis when full erection is achieved allows maintenance of the erection for periods of up to thirty minutes.

Surgical implants

Surgical implants are used when other forms of therapy are considered inappropriate or undesirable. By their nature, surgical implants rule out the possibility of the patient ever having a normal erection again. Erectile tissue in the penis is removed and replaced with silicone tubes that can be inflated from an internal reservoir and pump mechanism to allow them to become rigid. A satisfactory level of rigidity is achieved to allow intercourse, but the erect penis does not increase in diameter or length. This fact upsets some patients after surgery. Satisfaction rates are in the order of 80 per cent. It is an extremely expensive procedure, and the cost of the more commonly used device for this implant is over £2000 before any surgery.

Maintenance of erection is an increasing requirement of modern society. While not totally desirable in their make-up, these alternatives offer patients possibilities where none were available before.

TESTICULAR (TESTIS) CANCER

Knowledge about testicular cancer among the general public is extremely poor, despite the fact that this is the most common form of cancer in young men, with a peak incidence between fifteen and forty-five years of age. The risk is higher among men who have a history of undescended testes and in men with Down's Syndrome.

The tumour starts as a lump in the testis. From this initial site it spreads up into the abdomen and from there around the body. With early detection and treatment, however, there is an excellent chance of recovery.

The cure rate for testicular cancer in the early 1960s was extremely poor. With the introduction of a combination of chemotherapy using platinum and radical surgery, a complete turn-around has been achieved. Cure rates of the order of 97 per cent are now commonplace.

How can I identify testicular cancer?

The simplest way to identify testicular cancer is by regular self-examination of the testes. If you find any lump or swelling, you should always see your GP. The vast majority of lumps turn out to be benign cysts. These cysts are fluid-filled sacs lying around or near the testis. If there is any doubt or concern, you will be referred to the appropriate specialist for immediate assessment.

Testicular cancer is the most easily cured of all cancers, but early identification is the key to successful treatment.

Mr T E D McDermott FRCSI is a Consultant Urologist in the Meath Hospital and the Charlemont Clinic, Dublin. He has a particular interest in infertility, impotence and reconstructive surgery.

THE MENOPAUSE

DR MÁIRE MILNER

Menopause literally means the time when menstruation stops. The age of menopause, on average fifty-two years, has not varied for thousands of years.

Today, however, 'menopause' has come to mean the many problems that can occur, both at this time and in later years, and the subject has gained in importance as women are now living much longer. The average woman can expect to spend one third of her life after the menopause. More women than ever are looking for medical advice because of menstrual symptoms. Gynaecologist Dr Máire Milner explains how they can be helped.

WHY THE MENOPAUSE?

From the time of puberty, the ovary produces an egg each month (ovulation), with corresponding surges in the ovarian hormones, oestrogen and progesterone. With ageing, however, this occurs less regularly and with more difficulty until no further ovulations can take place. The levels of hormones drop, and no further periods occur. Oestrogen is the most important hormone, as deficiency during and after the menopause has many direct results.

Some women become menopausal for other reasons. The ovaries can be removed at surgery, or they can be damaged by chemotherapy or radiotherapy. A menopause between puberty and the age of forty is labelled 'premature'. It can occur spontaneously, with no cause found even after extensive tests.

A 'false' menopause can occur in athletes, when the prolonged heavy training and associated thinness can cause ovulation to cease. Anorexia nervosa likewise is accompanied by loss of menstruation. These are reversible conditions, but the lack of oestrogen, if prolonged, can cause long-term problems.

WHAT HAPPENS DURING MENOPAUSE?

Many women are fortunate in their experience of the menopause. Menstruation becomes more infrequent or stops abruptly. They have an occasional hot flush and encounter no real problems. However, others may suffer heavy, prolonged or irregular bleeding for several years before periods cease. This is an indication that the ovaries are having difficulty producing an egg, with its corresponding fluctuation in hormones, every month. Hot flushes or night sweats are the symptoms most women experience, but they are not necessarily the most distressing ones. Fatigue, an increase in anxiety/tension levels, panic attacks and palpitations can also be manifestations. Problems with passing water – burning and increased frequency – can result. Vaginal dryness can give rise to discomfort on making love.

In short, the menopause can affect women in many ways, although this is not to say that all problems are menopause-related, nor that all women require hormone replacement at this time.

THE BACKDROP TO MENOPAUSE

Middle-aged women have many problems to deal with. Ageing can bring ill-health for a women or her partner and there is consequently an increase in natural anxiety. Parents or other elderly relatives may become ill and increasingly dependent. Loss of a parent confronts us with our own mortality. Quite apart from grief, it signifies the passing of a generation.

It can be difficult to let go of children when they wish to make their own lives outside of the home. Feelings of dispensability are inevitable and encountered by most women at this time. However, the reverse is more often the case in Ireland. Children tend to marry at an older age than in other western countries and to live at home for longer. The end result is commonly a home, designed for a small family, becoming overcrowded with what has become a group of adults with differing habits and interests. Unemployment can further worsen matters to an intolerable level. This is a time when many couples feel that, having invested much of their lives in their offspring, they should be becoming free to enjoy more leisure time and each other. Having given for so long, however, most will continue to do so and not voice any objection.

In the years around the menopause, many personal and family stresses may feature, becoming important parts of the picture. The anxiety resulting from these problems can compound and indeed be confused with menopausal symptoms. On the other hand, true physical symptoms on top of other difficulties may be the straw that breaks the camel's back.

FEATURES OF THE MENOPAUSE

These can be divided into the symptoms that occur around this time and the much later problems of osteoporosis and cardiovascular disease.

Hot flushes and night sweats

These are the most common symptoms, affecting 70-80 per cent of women. A hot flush is a feeling of heat in the chest, neck and face, accompanied by redness and followed by profuse sweating.

Alcohol, tea, coffee, spicy food and being in company may all trigger flushes, which most women find embarrassing. Some may experience flushes every thirty minutes or more, others only occasionally. Flushes at night, or night sweats, are particularly distressing as they disturb sleep. The sweating may be so profuse that nightdress and bed clothes have to be changed. Some will sleep apart from their partner to minimise disturbance. All women with night sweats will feel tired and perform less well during the day, often with impaired concentration and memory. Though most women are free of these symptoms after two years, they may last for much longer – 25 per cent of women will suffer flushes and sweats five years after menopause.

Vaginal and bladder changes
The skin and glands in the vagina and bladder depend on an adequate oestrogen level to remain healthy. When this falls after the menopause, the vaginal skin thins and bleeds more easily. The glands produce less lubrication, leading to dry and painful lovemaking. Women not sexually active may experience an uncomfortable dry feeling in the vagina, often mistaken for 'thrush'. Women who have had a slight prolapse of the uterus may find the condition worsens as the muscles responsible for supporting the pelvic organs depend on oestrogen for strength and tone. Urinary symptoms of increased frequency and a burning sensation on passing water result from the water passage (urethra) and bladder becoming irritable. This mimics cystitis (or infection) and antibiotics can be mistakenly prescribed.

Period problems
As ovulation becomes more difficult with age, the resulting hormone imbalance can lead to a build-up of the lining of the womb (endometrium) and heavy, irregular periods. This can continue for several years before they eventually cease. However, as polyps, fibroids and cancer can cause similar problems, such a bleeding pattern should be reported as it requires investigation.

Psychological symptoms
Tiredness, loss of energy and interest, and poor concentration are

common complaints during the menopause. Anxiety, tension, forgetfulness and panic attacks also feature and are problems that can have a devastating impact on the quality of life. The situation may be made worse by night sweats, resulting in sleep disturbance. Curing them can result in a huge improvement in wellbeing by day. However, it is important not to attribute all ills to the menopause. Women must remember just how much they may have on their plate at this time, inside or outside the home. Anxiety and depression, if part of a problem that has already existed for years, and not linked to the menopause, will not improve with treatment for menopausal symptoms.

OSTEOPOROSIS

A progressive thinning or loss of density of bone occurs in everyone with age. This affects mainly the spine, forearms and hips. When it reaches a certain point, fractures may occur easily. Oestrogen is directly responsible for bone density, so low post-menopausal oestrogen levels render women much more suspectible than men to osteoporosis. Women especially at risk are those whose mother or aunts became stooped or suffered fractures; who have a thin or small frame; those whose menopause occurred prematurely; and smokers. Measuring the bone density with various X-ray or scanning techniques within a couple of years of the menopause is probably the best indicator of who will be at risk later.

CARDIOVASCULAR DISEASE

Coronary artery disease is the most common single cause of death in women in Ireland each year; over 90 per cent of deaths occur after the menopause. It is thought that oestrogen, through its effects on cholesterol and on blood vessel walls, protects women from heart diesease, but this protection is lost with the menopause. Studies have shown that hormone replacement therapy (HRT) can help decrease the risk of heart attack and stroke.

WHAT IS HORMONE REPLACEMENT THERAPY (HRT)?

The main component of this treatment is an oestrogen which closely resembles one's own hormone and 'replaces' this when low levels have been reached after the menopause. If a hysterectomy has been carried out, only oestrogen is necessary. However, if the womb (uterus) is intact, oestrogen taken alone can cause a progressive build-up of the endometrium (lining of the womb) which could lead to an overgrowth and perhaps eventually a cancer. Therefore, a second hormone, a progestogen similar to one's own progestogen, is added for part of each month and helps to counteract this build-up. When the progesterone is stopped, a period occurs. A new method has been developed whereby progestogen can be taken continuously with oestrogen so that build-up and bleeding are avoided. However, this is only suitable for women who are at least one year after menopause.

Forms of HRT

Oestrogen tablets are taken daily without a break. Progestogen is added in the same or a different tablet for ten to twelve days each month if bleeding is to occur. Tablets containing both hormones are available for a 'no bleed' regime.

Patches that release oestrogen continuously at a low but sufficient level are becoming popular. They require application twice per week and are particularly suitable for women who have had a hysterectomy. Otherwise, progestogen tablets need to be taken in conjunction each month. A patch containing both hormones is awaited.

Implants of oestrogen are inserted through a small nick in the skin of the thigh or abdomen under local anaesthetic. They are suitable for women after hysterectomy only. Symptoms recur generally three to six months later, when the process is repeated.

Vaginal creams are inserted with a fine tampon-like applicator over a two-week period. They release oestrogen to the vaginal skin and bladder base and are excellent for local symptoms. The relief generally lasts for several months. It can be repeated, and the short periods of use do not lead to endometrial build-up.

Pessaries of oestrogen have recently become available. They are preferred by some as less messy than creams.

Side-effects of HRT

Some nausea and breast tenderness initially are common with HRT. PMS-like symptoms of bloating, irritability etc may occur while taking progestogens. Bleeding at inappropriate times while taking the first couple of packets is common with all forms of HRT, particularly with continuous oestrogen/progestogen therapy. It is worth persevering with treatment, however, as many of these problems settle after a couple of months. Otherwise, changing to another brand may suit better. HRT does not cause weight gain. In fact, many women whose symptoms are relieved by treatment find they are able to diet successfully.

HRT lowers the risk of cancer of the uterus because of the regular bleeds and has no effect on ovarian or cervical cancer. Long-term therapy seems to be associated with some increase in risk of breast cancer, though it is unknown whether this is due to the fact that women on therapy have more frequent examinations and mammography. The increased risk has certainly not been observed with treatment periods of five years or less. HRT does not affect blood pressure nor does it cause clots.

Who cannot have HRT?

There is much confusion between the contraceptive pill and HRT. HRT comprises natural oestrogen, one sixth the strength of the pill, and yields levels in the blood lower than those the body is used to before menopause. Problems of blood pressure, clots and stroke which in the past were associated with high dose contraceptive pills are not relevant to HRT. Probably the only women who should not take HRT are those who have had breast cancer. Women with angina or those receiving treatment for high blood pressure may, in fact, be good candidates for HRT. Women who have had a thrombosis in the past may also be able to take it.

HRT – how long?

This depends on the reason for treatment. If taken for symptoms only, treatment can be discontinued after about two years, though some will need to recommence because of recurring symptoms. If HRT is taken because of a high risk of osteoporosis or cardiovascular disease, then a long-term period of five years or more should be considered to make a real impact on risk.

DIET, EXERCISE AND RECREATION

These are vital throughout all stages of life, not just at the menopause. Daily exercise and a balanced diet rich in calcium are important not only to prevent osteoporosis but to keep weight down and to maintain a reasonable level of cardiovascular fitness. Among the many negative effects of smoking are an earlier menopause and a greatly increased risk of both osteoporosis and cardiovascular disease. Smoking should therefore be stopped or kept to a minimum.

The benefits of taking time out for yourself on a regular basis cannot be over-emphasised. It is so easy for women to allow family stresses to submerge them, but getting other members of the family to help with an ageing relative or a disabled child can make all the difference. Acquiring a hobby, a part-time job or meeting friends once a week will ensure time outside the home. Many women cannot or will not do this, but it pays big dividends for personal development and makes for a higher level of appreciation by the family.

If there is any one piece of advice that is correct for all women approaching the menopause, it is to educate oneself as much as possible. There are many options for treatment and changes in lifestyle that will help not only to prolong life but to make that life both healthy and happy.

———————————

Dr Máire Milner MB, MRCOG is Assistant Master in the Rotunda Hospital, Dublin, where she runs a menopause clinic.

MOUTH AND TEETH

PROFESSOR D B SHANLEY

Your mouth is probably the most sensitive organ of your body. It is involved in many of your most sensitive functions – tasting, chewing, talking, breathing, kissing and facial expression. A pleasant smile with healthy gums and nice teeth is regarded as an essential part of looking good.

Professor Diarmuid Shanley, Dean of the Dublin Dental School, describes many of the conditions that can effect the mouth, from cold sores and bad breath to gum disease and toothache. He also advises on how you can get the best from your dentist . . .

The mouth is a wonderful example of the balance of nature. It is populated with billions of micro-organisms working in a so-called symbiotic relationship (we help them and they help us). As long as this balance is maintained, the mouth remains healthy. It is not easy to upset the balance, but it does happen when our resistance to disease is lowered or through unhealthy habits such as smoking, eating sugar too frequently or failing to keep the teeth sufficiently clean. Maintaining oral health is relatively simple. The two most common dental diseases are dental caries (dental decay) and periodontal disease (pyorrhoea or gum disease). Dental caries is the principal cause of tooth loss in all ages, while periodontal disease is a major cause of tooth loss in adults. Both are caused in different ways by dental plaque.

DENTAL PLAQUE

Dental (bacterial) plaque accumulates around the necks of the teeth and in between the teeth where it is most inaccessible and protected from the effects of saliva and brushing. It also deposits itself on any artificial appliances in the mouth, such as bridges, dentures etc. Plaque is a collection of millions of bacteria stuck to the tooth surface in a developing and highly organised micro-colony. Plaque is virtually invisible, but we can sometimes feel it with our tongue as a furry or coarse feeling on the enamel of our teeth.

PLAQUE AND DECAY

Plaque absorbs sugar from food, and bacteria turn it into an acid. Some bacteria use the sugar to build a sticky scaffolding which helps bacteria to stick both to each other and to the tooth's surface. Saliva is unable to wash it away. Within twenty minutes of taking sugar, the bacterial acid is sufficiently strong to demineralise (dissolve) tooth enamel. The more frequently we take sugar, the more frequently the enamel is attacked by acid, and the more likely it is that a cavity will develop. The less frequently we eat sugar, the better. Soft drinks, ice cream, sweets and biscuits are particularly destructive to teeth because of their high sugar content. Given their popularity, it is very important to establish good dietary habits in infants and young children.

If a child is given sweets, they should be eaten all at once. This would only cause one acid attack. If, however, they are eaten one by one during the day, this could mean as many as twenty acid attacks. Better still, children should be encouraged to brush their teeth with a toothpaste containing fluoride after eating sweets, as this helps to reverse the acid destruction.

PLAQUE AND GUM DISEASE

Periodontal disease (gum disease) begins as inflammation in the gum margins at the neck of the tooth. It occurs more commonly between the teeth where it is not easy to remove plaque. Plaque bacteria excrete toxic substances which irritate the gum margin. There is usually a balance between the resistance of the host (ourselves) and the destructive elements of plaque. This battle continues throughout our lifetime. It can, however, cause destruction of the bone under the gum which supports the teeth. Teeth may become loose as a consequence. The more effectively we remove plaque, the more we tip the balance towards healthy gums.

The most important sign of early gum disease is bleeding from the gums, which may first be noticed as traces of blood on your toothbrush. Healthy gums should not bleed. If they do, you have gum disease. If your dentist tells you that it is quite normal to have bleeding gums, ask for a second opinion. Constant bad breath is also a common sign of the problem. Another sign of gum disease is when adults develop new spaces between their teeth, but the condition is usually advanced when this happens.

DENTAL CALCULUS

If plaque is left on the tooth surface, it can become calcified and turn into calculus (tartar). Tartar can also form below the margin of the gums when they are inflamed. It has a rough surface which is seething with micro-organisms, adding to the irritation of the gums and periodontal tissues (tissues around and supporting the teeth).

HYGIENE AND PREVENTION

The mouth has its own natural cleansing mechanism. The constant movement of the tissues inside the mouth combines with a constant flow of saliva. When you wake up in the morning, your mouth can be dry and have a bad taste, and your breath can smell (halitosis) because the normal cleansing mechanisms virtually cease during sleep. Those who have had diseases or injuries that affect the salivary glands or that prevent normal movement will notice that the mouth can become uncomfortably dry. In such circumstances, plaque accumulates on the teeth very rapidly.

We supplement the mouth's highly effective self-cleaning process with our own 'artificial' oral hygiene. Most people do not clean their teeth properly, spending less than one minute brushing their teeth. Inevitably, the same parts are missed each time. These are the parts where disease can begin. Nature cleans the top two-thirds of the crowns of the teeth (the exposed parts). So we need to concentrate on the necks of the teeth (at the gum margins) and the areas in between the teeth.

Each tooth has four or five surfaces that need to be cleaned properly at least once a day and brushed reasonably well on another one or two occasions, if possible. Remember – you are attempting to remove or scrape away a tenacious film of bacteria from each surface without damaging the gum tissue.

Disclosing tablets or food dyes which stain plaque can be used every week or so to check brushing technique. Use these products after you have cleaned your teeth. Then look in a mirror, in good light, to see what parts you have missed. Most people fail to clean the inside of the back teeth and in between the back teeth.

Cleaning between the teeth is both the most difficult and the most important part of oral hygiene. For this, dental floss is best. It requires both patience and dexterity. If you have neither of these attributes, you can use the tip of the bristles on your toothbrush, poking it between your teeth. Make sure it is worked gently into the spaces between all of the teeth, particularly those in the back of your mouth. Wooden points are also easy to use and useful for cleaning between the teeth and around the necks of the teeth. For those with large spaces between their teeth, special interproximal brushes are excellent and available in your chemist's shop.

Despite all their claims, most well-known toothpastes are more or less the same. Use a short-headed, medium, nylon-tufted toothbrush with a straight handle and without too many fancy extras. Do not use a hard toothbrush, as this causes excessive wear of the enamel of the teeth and damages the gums. Do not use toothpastes that are too harsh, such as 'smoker's' toothpaste.

Use either a vibratory method or a small circular movement with your toothbrush, pointing the bristles in under the margin of the gum both inside and outside, cleaning only two teeth at a time. In order for fluoride, anti-plaque and anti-calculus agents in toothpaste to have any effect, it must be left in the mouth for at least a minute before spitting out.

GUM RECESSION

Most adults with healthy mouths have some degree of gum recession (the teeth begin to look longer), and this is not usually a problem. However, it can be excessive in those who brush their teeth too vigorously, particularly if a hard toothbrush is used. When a root is exposed as a result of recession, it can become sensitive, particularly if it is not kept clean. Fluoride reduces sensitivity. Some toothpastes have desensitising agents which may also help. There are also surgical methods to cover exposed roots of teeth, including transplantation of gum tissue. The benefits of such surgery are debatable. Ask your dentist for advice.

FLUORIDE

Fluoride is a naturally occurring trace element in water. Where it occurs, it was discovered that people had significantly less dental

185

decay. Fluoride increases the strength of the enamel crystals in the teeth. It helps re-mineralise or repair the destruction of enamel by acid attack. It has anti-bacterial effects and it may delay the formation of plaque.

In Ireland, fluoride has been added to the drinking water for nearly thirty years. At a level of one part per million, it has had a dramatic effect on improving dental health. Despite repeated scare reports on potential hazards of fluoride, it is a safe and effective way of reducing dental caries and is the most widely researched public health measure.

Unfortunately, one-third of the people in Ireland do not have fluoride in their drinking water. If that is the case in your area, consult your dentist about using fluoride supplements. If your drinking water is fluoridated do not use fluoride supplements. Excessive fluoride can lead to staining of the enamel which initially appears as white spots. It can be more severe with higher dosages and can cause mottling or brown pitting of enamel.

ORTHODONTICS

Orthodontic treatment is almost invariably carried out for purposes of appearance. It is difficult to understand why it costs so much in Ireland. Except in exceptional cases, it has no beneficial effect in preventing the common dental diseases. Nature never intended us to have perfectly symmetrical teeth, and some people have lost their own natural facial characteristics from over-zealous orthodontic treatment. Avoid it if at all possible. Your dentist will advise you. It is, of course, difficult to dissuade children or their parents once they are convinced that they need orthodontics. Of course, it is necessary for those with serious occlusal problems (faulty bite), but in Ireland, those who most need it do not necessarily receive it.

PARTIAL (REMOVABLE) AND FULL DENTURES

If a permanent tooth is extracted or lost, it is not always necessary to have it replaced. Replacement prostheses (ie bridges or dentures) must be made and fitted to the highest technical and biological standards. Otherwise they can do more harm than good. Artificial teeth interfere with the natural cleansing activities of the mouth and can encourage more plaque deposition. Unless there are very good reasons for a partial denture or a bridge, and they are usually cosmetic reasons, do not embark on an expensive course of treatment. Discuss the pros and cons with your dentist.

Denture hygiene is extremely important, particularly in the case of partial dentures, and it is essential to follow the instructions of your dentist. If you have not been given any, you should ask.

Most people are embarrassed to be seen without their dentures. However, it is essential to remove dentures before going to sleep in order to allow the tissues of the mouth to remain healthy. Imagine what would happen to your feet if you left your shoes on all the time!

PAIN AND TOOTHACHE

Toothache is one of the most common reasons for seeing the dentist, yet most dental diseases, including dental decay and abscesses, do not usually cause pain. This gives an indication of how much dental disease remains undiscovered.

The most common cause of toothache is inflammation of the pulp of the tooth. This is usually because of a deep carious cavity (decay). It can also occur following the placement of a deep filling which can irritate the pulp. Toothache may start as sensitivity to cold drinks. As time goes on, acute (rapid onset) inflammation becomes chronic and sometimes there is severe pain. The pulp may eventually die. The dead tooth discolours and becomes grey. A similar problem can occur following a sharp, sudden blow to a tooth which tears or permanently damages the delicate blood vessels that supply each tooth.

The dead tooth pulp tissue may subsequently become infected, which may lead to abscess formation (the tooth becomes sensitive to touch). An abscess is a collection of pus and this may spread. Before antibiotics, some dental abscesses had fatal consequences. Your dentist can bring relief by extracting the tooth or by incising directly into the abscess to drain the pus. The best way is to drain the abscess through the tooth (root canal or endodontic treatment). The empty chamber of the tooth is then filled with an inert material.

DISCOLOURED TEETH

Teeth vary in shade from a very bright, almost white colour which is quite unusual, to shades of yellow or grey. As we get older, our teeth become stained. Teeth can be stained from external deposits or by internal sources such as antibiotics (tetracyclines) taken during tooth formation.

Teeth that are stained can be bleached by the dentist. When that is not possible, there are different methods to restore the tooth's appearance. For example, the tooth can be coated with new materials, or a fine ceramic film can be placed on the discoloured tooth as a veneer.

External stains

The most common cause of tooth staining is smoking. Red wine, some mouthwashes and black tea also stain teeth. Ageing results in a darker shade of tooth. Most toothpastes help remove stains with ordinary toothbrushing. Stains can be easily removed by your dentist. There are also new bleaching toothpastes which are effective but expensive.

COLD SORES (HERPES SIMPLEX)

Some people are afflicted by cold sores on the lips more frequently than others. The cold sore is due to the *Herpes simplex* virus. Those who are susceptible to this virus may develop the condition when their resistance is lowered, following illness or exposure to too much sunlight. A cold sore begins with a tingly or itchy sensation, followed by the development of a cluster of small blisters called vesicles. The small vesicles rupture and a cold sore is formed. Depending on the size of the blistering and ulceration, it can take from five to ten days to heal.

There are anti-viral ointments such as Zovirax which are effective if they are applied when the area is first itchy or tingling. Once the ulcer has formed, however, they are of little use. The ointment must be applied for three or four days. It has a short shelf life, so used tubes should be replaced when a new cold sore begins to develop.

Cold sores may be highly infective and you should be careful to avoid passing them to others. Young children who have not previously been exposed to the *Herpes simplex* virus can develop quite severe generalised conditions and become very ill. Anyone who is debilitated should be particularly careful to avoid close contact with people with cold sores. If you are susceptible, be careful of exposure to excessive sunlight, and use a sunblock on the lips.

MOUTH ULCERS

The most common form of mouth ulcer is aphthous ulceration, sometimes called canker sores. Aphthous ulcers are grey, shallow ulcers with red borders, and are particularly sore for the first few days. It takes about seven to ten days before healing is complete. In the vast majority of cases, the cause of these ulcers is unknown (idiopathic).

Aphthous ulcers may increase in frequency during menstruation or times of stress. They can be caused by local physical irritants, such as a sharp edge on a tooth or a filling, or damage from a toothbrush. Elimination of roughness and sharp edges can bring relief. This, together with good oral hygiene, is usually the first treatment provided by the dentist. Ulceration can be reduced in frequency and severity with good oral hygiene and a mouthwash such as Corsodyl.

Aphthous ulceration is also associated with certain vitamin deficiencies and gastrointestinal disorders. It is advisable to consult your dentist if you suffer from this problem. He or she will then refer you, if necessary, for further investigation.

An ulcer that lasts for more than two weeks may be more

serious even if it is painless. Your dentist or doctor should identify the cause of such an ulcer.

ORAL CANCER

Ireland has a high incidence of oral cancer, particularly cancer of the lip. Oral cancer is one of the more serious cancers and is linked directly to smoking, particularly when combined with high levels of alcohol consumption. If you want to avoid this dreadful condition, stop smoking. Again, excessive sunlight causes skin and lip cancer, so protect yourself with a sun block.

IMPACTED WISDOM TEETH

There are usually thirty-two teeth in the mouth. Sometimes there is not enough room for all of them to erupt and the teeth which erupt last, the third molars (wisdom teeth), are most likely to be crowded out and become impacted or blocked. It may be necessary to have these removed if they are infected or impacted. This problem usually affects teenagers and young adults.

If there is inflammation (pericoronitis) and pain of the gum over an impacted wisdom tooth, rinsing with hot water and salt (a teaspoon in a glass of water) may help to drain pus and ease the pain. Antibiotics are usually prescribed to reduce acute infection. The tooth may need to be removed when the infection subsides.

The roots of the lower wisdom teeth are close to two nerves that provide sensation to the lower lip and the tongue. Both nerves are at risk of damage from surgery, even from the most talented dental or oral surgeon, when wisdom teeth are being removed. Your dentist will advise you of the likelihood of this problem prior to surgery.

CROWNS AND BRIDGES

A crown is used to rebuild a badly broken-down tooth. It is made from gold, procelain or a mixture of both. The dentist first files about a millimetre from the tooth and then takes an impression of the tooth that needs to be restored. This is sent to a dental technician who makes the crown. The crown, which is a hollow shell, is then cemented into place over the prepared tooth.

A crown can also be part of a bridge. When a tooth is lost, the space can be repaired with a false tooth attached to a crown on either side. Crowns can be very expensive.

IMPLANTS

Implants are not new. In the seventeeth and eighteenth centuries, it was not uncommon for the wealthy to have their own bad teeth removed and healthy teeth implanted from the less-well-off who were paid for this unethical practice. The only factor in common with modern implant techniques is that it continues to be a solution for the wealthy. Implants are extremely expensive, so be sure to discuss the costs before embarking on a course of treatment. The VHI covers only part of the costs of a very expensive procedure for those who otherwise are unable to wear full lower dentures.

Dental implants are done in stages. An incision is made to expose the bone into which fine holes are drilled. Then, metal implants are placed into these holes. After a time, these integrate with the bone of the jaw. A second surgical procedure is usually necessary to re-expose the implanted artificial roots. Individual teeth, groups of teeth, or full replacements for all teeth are then secured into the implants with tiny screws.

MERCURY IN AMALGAM

The most commonly used dental filling material is called dental amalgam, which contains mercury. Mercury is a toxic material and there has been concern about its use in fillings. Amalgam has been in use for over a century. There is little evidence that it has harmful effects, except in a small number of patients in whom the amalgam irritates the mucosa (the lining) of the mouth. Dental amalgam continues to be the best filling material for the back teeth because it is cheap, easy to work with, and has stood the test of time. There is no justification for the replacement of amalgam fillings with white fillings because of fears of mercury poisoning. As yet, there is no satisfactory white filling material that can be used as effectively in the back teeth.

AIDS, HIV INFECTION AND THE DENTIST

Patients who become infected with the HIV virus may first show signs of the infection in their mouth. The HIV virus causes major disruption of the normal defence mechanisms. What might have been a simple problem such as a mouth ulcer in a healthy person can present major complications for the HIV-infected patient. It is essential for those who have the virus to maintain strict oral hygiene and to attend for regular dental and oral care to avoid such complications. In those who are terminally ill with AIDS, oral and dental infections can become extremely difficult to control and may cause severe discomfort.

Many people are worried about the dangers of being infected with the HIV virus by their dentist. These fears are understandable, but in fact there has only been one reported case of a dentist infecting patients. There have been no reported cases of dentists or dental nurses being infected by patients. Nevertheless, dentists are now taking much greater precautions to control cross-infection in their surgeries because of AIDS and Hepatitis B, which is more easily transmitted. Instruments should be thoroughly sterilised between patients and this requires the use of a modern autoclave (sterilising unit). This works like a pressure cooker and is the most practical and efffective way of killing all forms of micro-organisms.

Dentists should use rubber gloves. This not only protects the patient from any bacteria or viruses on the dentist's hands but also protects the dentist from the patient's micro-organisms. Masks are worn for the same purpose. Dentists now wear glasses to protect their eyes from splashes and spray from the patient's mouth which can be contaminated with dangerous viruses.

All instruments, including the delicate dental drill, must be autoclaved between patients. If you are in any doubt about whether or not your dentist carries out these basic sterilising precautions, simply ask and you will be told.

YOU AND YOUR DENTIST

It is important to adopt a regular pattern of visiting your dentist. Six-monthly visits are recommended for children, for those who are very susceptible to dental disease and for those who have had extensive dental treatment. Once a year is probably sufficient for most adults. A good dentist will not overtreat and is in the best position to advise on the frequency of recall visits.

Private dental treatment is a contract between the patient and the dentist. You should discuss the cost of each treatment in advance with your dentist. You should be made aware of the benefits of that treatment and the consequences of not having such treatment carried out. You should also be informed of the potential deleterious consequences of treatment. You should then be able to make an informed judgement as to whether or not you wish to have the recommended treatment.

A good dentist is one who:

• is concerned with promoting health and prevention;

• minimises the amount of treatment a patient requires to maintain oral health;

• is sympathetic and practical;

• provides the most effective care for the least cost and inconvenience;

• listens to your concerns before starting treatment.

Word of mouth is important in judging a dentist. Avoid dentists who:

• recommend unnecessary expensive treatments (if the charges seem overly expensive, you have the right to go to another dentist for a second opinion);

• do not emphasise prevention, particularly for children;

• do not emphasise the significance of frequent sugar consumption;

• do not carry out a careful examination of the whole mouth;

• do not sterilise instruments properly – instruments need to be sterilised in an autoclave (like a pressure pot), not in an old-fashioned boiler;

- do not change gloves between patients;
- are overly critical of other dentists' work;
- do not have their home telephone number in the telephone book in case of emergencies.

A dentist who carries out complicated, extensive and expensive treatment is not necessarily a good dentist. It is the effective and simple maintenance of health that is important, not high technology.

FEAR OF THE DENTIST

Many people are afraid of going to the dentist. Such fear is understandable. Acceptance of the fact that one is fearful is the first step in overcoming it. All dentists are familiar with the problem and are used to dealing with it. In extreme cases, methods such as general anaesthesia, sedation and hypnosis are employed to overcome the patient's fear. Don't be ashamed to tell your dentist of your fears or of any past experience that caused anxiety. You are assured of a sympathetic ear from almost all dentists.

Diarmuid Shanley MA, MSCD, FFDRCSI, FDSRCSED, FTCD is Professor of Oral Health at Trinity College, Dublin, a Consultant Periodontologist, and Dean of Dental Affairs at the Dublin Dental School and Hospital.

PAIN

PROFESSOR C A O'BOYLE

People vary enormously in the way they react to pain. What seems like a minor discomfort to one person may be absolute agony for someone else. Understanding the mechanism of pain may in itself help us to cope with it better.

Psychologist Professor Ciaran O'Boyle explains what pain is, how it affects us and what can be done to control it. He also includes instructions for a simple relaxation therapy that can help not only in pain relief, but also in reducing stress . . .

THE PUZZLE OF PAIN

Most people think that pain is always the result of physical injury and that there is a direct link between the amount of pain experienced and the extent of physical injury. A pin-prick to the finger causes little pain, whereas a door slammed on that same finger causes excruciating pain. People think that when an injury occurs, the nerves carry information directly to the brain and that the pain experienced is in direct proportion to the amount of the injury. This, however, cannot be the full story. Sportsmen and women get hurt on the playing field and, in the heat of the game, get up and carry on. Two thirds of soldiers seriously wounded in battle, one fifth of patients undergoing major surgery and about a third of patients injured in accidents report feeling little or no pain for hours, even days after the injury. In contrast, individuals who suffer from a condition called hyperalgesia experience the most excruciating pain even when their skin is gently rubbed. Anyone who has ever passed a kidney stone knows the pain that such a tiny object can cause. Being tired, anxious or depressed can make pain worse, while being relaxed or concentrating on something else can lessen pain. To understand this complicated relationship between injury and pain, some of the characteristics of pain must be considered.

TYPES OF PAIN

Pain is usually classified into two major types, acute and chronic. Acute pain is relatively short-lived and can range from the fairly minor pain of a toothache or a headache to the agony of a heart attack. It usually lasts only as long as the condition that is causing it and responds well to treatment. Such pain causes fear and anxiety and the sufferer is usually preoccupied with both the pain and its consequences. Acute pain acts as a warning to the individual to seek the best means of treatment and recovery. Certain types of nerves called Aô fibres conduct this type of pain information very rapidly from the site of injury to the brain.

The importance of acute pain as a warning signal is obvious when one considers cases of individuals who are born without the ability to feel pain. Such people are normal in every way, except that they cannot feel pain. This might seem like a great advantage, but the consequences are usually serious. One patient died as a result of massive infections resulting from inflammation in her joints. This was caused by damage due to her failure to shift her weight when standing for long periods or to turn over during her sleep. Another patient with an acute appendicitis was saved by the quick thinking of her doctor who realised what her description of 'a tight feeling' meant. Others scar their mouths by drinking scalding beverages or burn other parts of their bodies unknowingly. Acute pain, therefore, plays an important role in survival by acting as a warning system. However, there is another type of pain, chronic pain, which appears to be of little or no value.

One of the major advances in medicine has been the realisation that chronic pain is a distinct entity, different from acute pain. It persists after healing has occurred, long after the pain serves any useful function and when it is no longer simply a symptom of injury or disease. Unlike acute pain, chronic pain has no biological value and is a most disabling condition. It affects the whole person, physically, psychologically, emotionally and spiritually. It is impossible to predict when it will end; it often gets worse rather than better. It lacks any positive meaning and frequently expands to fill the person's whole attention and isolates him or her from the world around them. Patients experience helplessness, hopelessness and despair. Severe depression and anger are common. The patient's behaviour also changes. He or she feels trapped and fully occupied by the pain. It seem endless. One patient remarked, 'It is always three o'clock in the morning.' Chronic pain is conducted to the brain along nerves called c-fibres which are different from the Aô fibres that are involved in acute pain.

THE GATE-CONTROL THEORY OF PAIN

In the 1960s, two researchers proposed a theory that has revolutionised the understanding and treatment of pain. This was

THE CHECK UP GUIDE TO GOOD HEALTH

called the Gate-Control Theory because it proposed that information coming from an injured area must pass through a type of gate in the spinal cord on its way to the brain. If the gate is open, the nerve impulses pass through and the person experiences pain. However, if the gate is closed, no information can pass, so that even a major injury will not be experienced as painful. The important factors are, therefore, those that determine whether the gate is open or closed.

Conditions that open the pain gate

Physical conditions
    Extent of the injury
    Inappropriate activity level such as running with severe arthritis

---

Emotional conditions
    Anxiety and worry
    Tension
    Depression

Mental conditions
    Focusing on the pain
    Boredom; little involvement in life activities

Conditions that close the pain gate

Physical conditions
    Medication
    Heat, massage

Emotional conditions
    Positive emotions such as happiness or optimism
    Relaxation
    Rest

Mental conditions
    Intense concentration or distraction
    Involvement and interest in life activities

Research has shown that three factors are important in controlling the gate. First, the amount of energy in the nerves that send pain messages is important. The greater the injury, the greater will be the energy in the pain nerves. This will tend to open the gate. The second important factor is that activity in other nerves, called sensory-motor nerves, tends to close the gate. If you hit your finger with a hammer, you will probably jump up and down, shaking your hand. You may also utter certain words and phrases to lend colour to the situation. Shaking your hand, sucking or rubbing the sore finger stimulates the sensory nerves which will tend to close the gate so that the information in the pain nerves finds it more difficult to get through to the brain. Massage and heat have the same effect, as do techniques such as acupuncture.

The third important factor is the brain itself. The brain can open or close the gate. If we are anxious, depressed, unhappy or concentrating on our pain, this will open the gate and let more of the pain information through to the brain. The result will be increased pain. If we are relaxed, optimistic or concentrating deeply on something other than the pain, this will tend to close the gate and we will feel less pain. This probably explains the effects of hypnosis and trance states in which people can tolerate severe pain.

It is clear from the Gate-Control Theory that there are a number of approaches that can be used in treating pain. The major aim is to use all possible means to close the gate.

COMMUNICATION OF PAIN

Another related but crucial problem in dealing with pain is that of communication. Pain is a private, personal experience which is common to all of us yet unique to each of us. It means very different things to different people. Pain is influenced by the context in which it occurs, its meaning for the individual, the person's previous experience of it and the amount of attention paid to it. People from very different backgrounds tend to use the same comparisons to familiar objects. Pain is 'like a knife';

'hammers pounding inside my head'; 'like a red hot-poker'. Other common descriptions are words such as dull, sharp, aching, throbbing, burning.

One of the major problems in controlling pain is that, being a very personal experience, it is difficult to communicate. Doctors are only coming to realise the importance of providing their patients with scales and questionnaires that help them to communicate exactly what their pain is like.

One simple technique for communicating about pain is called the visual analogue scale. This is a line anchored at either end respectively by the phrases 'No pain' and 'Pain as bad as it could possibly be'.

No pain	_____	Pain as bad as it could possibly be

The person places a mark on the line at a point corresponding to their present level of pain. This strategy can be used repeatedly in pain diaries by having the patient make such a rating every hour. This provides useful information about the pattern of pain and what makes it worse. For patients suffering from chronic pain, making and completing such a diary can provide very useful information for themselves and their doctors.

PAIN RELIEF AND MANAGEMENT

Doctors are recognising that there are many approaches to pain relief and management, and that the best approach is to use a number of approaches together. A good example of this is ante-natal training for childbirth. Here, a number of techniques are combined to ensure that labour is as free of pain as possible. Expectant mothers and their partners are taught how to focus on and control their breathing and how to use this technique to relax. They are provided with information on childbirth in order to reduce the stress that normally accompanies unfamiliar events. In addition, they may choose to have an epidural anaesthetic. This involves the injection of an anaesthetic drug into the fluid surrounding the spinal cord so that pain messages are prevented from reaching the brain. This is an example of combining psychological (information, relaxation, distraction) and pharmacological (anaesthetic) techniques.

Another important example of pain relief and management is in preparing patients for surgery. In 1964, a group of doctors in the US showed the importance of psychological preparation in reducing pain after operations. They divided patients who were having major surgery into two groups. One group was treated using normal hospital practice, while the second was psychologically prepared before the operation. They were told about the type and level of pain they would be likely to experience after the operation and were reassured that such pain was normal and would decrease over time. They were taught a relaxation technique and shown how to breathe and move without putting strain on the surgical wound. The prepared group experienced significantly less pain after surgery, required about half the dose of pain-killers and could be discharged from hospital two days sooner, on average, than the non-prepared group. Therefore, it makes good sense to prepare yourself if you are going to have an operation, by finding out as much as you can in advance and learning a few simple relaxation techniques.

PAIN-KILLERS

Pain-killing drugs or analgesics are widely used in our society. There are three major types:
- non-steroidal anti-inflammatory drugs called NSAIDs, such as aspirin
- local anaesthetics
- morphine-like drugs called narcotic analgesics.

NSAIDs which include aspirin, paracetamol and ibuprofen are among the most widely used of all drugs and are bought in their millions every year. These drugs have three actions: they lower raised temperature; they reduce certain types of pain; they decrease inflammation. They act mainly by inhibiting the production of pain-producing substances in the body.

Local anaesthetics are drugs such as those that are used by dentists. They block pain by preventing the pain messages from travelling along nerves to the brain. These are also the drugs that are used in epidural anaesthesia for preventing the pain associated with childbirth.

The narcotic analgesics such as morphine are powerful drugs which act on the brain and spinal cord to reduce pain. A problem with this class of drugs, which includes heroin, is that they can be addictive and can interfere with breathing. However, it has become clear that these are much less serious problems in patients with chronic pain.

PATIENT-CONTROLLED ANALGESIA

Most people will take an aspirin to relieve a headache. This is an example of patient-controlled analgesia. It has the advantage of allowing the individual to judge whether the drug is needed, how much is needed and whether it is effective or not. Allowing hospital patients to control their own pain medication is becoming more common for certain types of pain. Following surgery, for example, patients would usually be given pain-killers at regular intervals, according to their doctors' instructions. Now, however, there is a device consisting of a pump attached to a needle in a vein which will allow patients to take the pain-killer whenever they feel they need it. The pump has controls that prevent the patient from delivering too much of the drug at any one time. It has been found that patients using this method generally use lower doses of analgesics than when the drug is prescribed and administered in the traditional manner.

PSYCHOLOGICAL APPROACHES TO
PAIN MANAGEMENT

The brain plays a crucial role in the perception of pain. Psychological factors such as previous experience, attention, meaning and the context in which the pain occurs are all important factors in the experience of pain. Because of this, psychological techniques can play a useful role in the management of relatively mild or moderate pain. In treatment, the concern should be not the pain the patient has, but rather the patient with the pain. If doctors and nurses set about the relief of pain and discomfort with sincerity and competence, their intention alone often brings relief. There are, however, psychological techniques that the patient can use. These include distraction, relaxation and imagery.

Distraction

Have you ever noticed that a doctor or a nurse usually chats with you when giving you an injection or performing a painful procedure? Have you ever found yourself counting the tiles on the dentist's ceiling when he is drilling? If you suffer from chronic pain, have you noticed that listening to the radio, watching a favourite TV programme, knitting or having someone to talk to all reduce your pain? A rather bizarre example of distraction is that of a patient who suffered such severe pain that the only way she could help herself was by banging her head on the floor. 'It gives me another pain to think about,' she explained. These are all examples of distraction. By focusing one's attention on something other than the pain, the pain itself can be reduced.

Relaxation

Stress can make most types of pain worse. It can even cause certain types of pain such as headache, migraine and muscular pain. Relaxation is useful in reducing such pain. It not only decreases muscle tension and spasm but also assists patients to rest and sleep better. Relaxation techniques are also forms of distraction which can help take the person's mind off the pain.

Imagery

When children are about to receive an injection, their parents will often say something such as, 'It'll be easier if you think about something pleasant, like the time we went on holidays'. Non-pain imagery is a technique whereby the person tries to alleviate discomfort by conjuring up a mental scene that is unrelated to or incompatible with the pain. The best images are those that are pleasant and that involve all the senses. If elements of the image can be seen, heard, smelled, touched and tasted, it is more likely to be effective in reducing pain. An example is imagining a beach, the sight and smell of the water, the sound of the breeze and the waves lapping at the shore, the warm grainy feel of the sand. Imagery is often used along with relaxation to induce a state that is incompatible with pain. The technique can include intense concentration exercises such as imagining oneself going through drawers or cupboards, clearing out the attic, sewing specific stitches, reading specific books and so on.

PAIN IN TERMINAL ILLNESS

In the past, many patients with a terminal illness such as cancer had to endure a great deal of pain. Now, there is much that can be done to help such patients and to relieve their suffering. The hospice movement, which was founded in Ireland, is a worldwide movement that places emphasis on care for those for whom cure is not feasible. Importance is placed on controlling symptoms, especially pain, to ensure that the quality of life that remains is maximised. The aim is to anticipate and prevent symptoms rather than waiting for them to arise and then treating them. The hospice also concerns itself with the psychological and spiritual needs of patients and their families. The hospice movement has recently been extended into the community through the development of home-care teams. These usually consist of specially trained doctors and nurses who, in consultation with the general practitioner, ensure that patients who are being cared for at home are free from pain and have the level of total care that meets their needs. One terminally ill patient defined the prime purpose of the hospice as follows: 'I am a traveller on the journey from one life to the next, and I need a place where I can be welcomed and looked after and cared for and be myself on that journey.'

A SIMPLE RELAXATION TECHNIQUE

Step 1: Find a quiet, comfortable place where you will not be disturbed.

Step 2: Sit or lie in a comfortable position.

Step 3: Close your eyes and begin to check your body for tension. Start with your feet. Note any tension and relax the muscles of your feet. Move up to your calves, your hips, bottom. Let your stomach sag. Relax your chest and arms. Let your hands fall open. Let your shoulders drop. Let the expression go from your face.

Step 4: Become aware of your breathing. Don't try to change your breathing but bring all your attention to focus on your breathing. Concentrate only on your breathing. Your mind will wander. Don't let this bother you. Bring your attention passively back to your breathing. With practice over a few weeks, you should be able to keep your mind clear of everything but your breathing. Now each time you breathe out, say the word 'calm' quietly to yourself. Continue for about twenty minutes. You may open your eyes to check the time but do not use an alarm. When you finish, sit quietly for several minutes, at first with closed eyes and later with open eyes.

Step 5: Do this for about twenty minutes every day and after a week or so you should see results. Don't worry about whether you are successful in achieving a deep level of relaxation. Maintain a passive attitude and allow relaxation to occur at its own pace. You should be able to relax much more quickly. At times when you find yourself getting upset, anxious or angry, simply practise your technique.

Some don'ts

Don't do your relaxation for about two hours after eating.

Don't set an alarm clock to tell you when your relaxation time is up.

Don't stand up too suddenly after relaxation.

Professor C A O'Boyle BSc, PhD, Reg Psychol (APsSI), CPsychol (AFBPsS) is Professor of Psychology at the Medical School of the Royal College of Surgeons in Ireland. He is also qualified as a pharmacologist and has a particular interest in the areas of stress and pain.

PREMENSTRUAL SYNDROME

DR VALERIE DONNELLY

Most women are aware of the changes that take place in their own bodies each month. Some breast discomfort, bloating and mood changes are considered a normal part of life. However, there are women who have severe symptoms which occur on a monthly basis and disappear at the start of a period. Premenstrual syndrome (PMS) is a very real phenomenon and can pose huge problems for sufferers. It is only in the fairly recent past that the medical profession has taken the condition seriously.

Gynaecologist Dr Valerie Donnelly explains how you can identify whether or not you have PMS. She offers practical and sensible advice about what you can do to help yourself and when you should seek medical help . . .

WHAT IS PMS?

In 1931, Dr R H T Frank coined the term 'premenstrual tension'. Despite over sixty years of scientific research, the causes of the condition and the best ways to treat it are still unclear.

PMS affects not only the sufferer herself – it also affects her performance at work and at home. It affects her relationship with her partner, her functioning as a mother and her social life.

It is not known how many women in Ireland suffer from PMS but it is estimated that approximately 10 per cent are affected.

PMS is the recurrence of symptoms in the second half of the monthly cycle. The symptoms abate once the period has started and during the first half of the next cycle. It is the timing of these symptoms, not the symptoms themselves, that is the most important feature, since the various symptoms can occur in other conditions, in both men and women. So the distinguishing feature of PMS is the cyclical timing of the symptoms.

WHO GETS PMS?

Every woman from puberty to menopause has a menstrual cycle and can therefore suffer from PMS. A woman can suffer from it at any stage. PMS is often triggered by a major event such as having a baby, starting or stopping the oral contraceptive pill, a family death or a hysterectomy. Hysterectomy patients wonder how they could be suffering from PMS, having had their womb removed. However, if the ovaries have been left behind, PMS can still occur.

Women of any age can get PMS, though it more commonly occurs between the ages of thirty-five and forty-five, after which the symptoms generally ease off. This does not happen in all cases, although it is a general rule. Why PMS should affect women particularly at this stage is not clear. It is thought that at this time, one's reproductive years are nearing an end, and even though the woman herself may have completed her family and has no wish for more children, her body continues to ovulate.

When a teenager suffers from severe PMS, she may feel quite depressed at the possibility of having the condition for the rest of her reproductive years. This, however, is not the case, as in most women, PMS comes and goes and is not static.

PMS clinics often report that there is a higher proportion of women attending with phobias, psychiatric disorders and alcohol abuse than in other comparative groups. It is certain that depressed patients or those with other psychiatric conditions have premenstrual exacerbation of their symptoms. A woman can suffer from depression and PMS at the same time. For this reason, the diagnosis is very important and should be made by a qualified doctor.

Some people have suggested that PMS is associated with a particular personality type, but many women who suffer from severe PMS have entirely normal personalities; daughters of women who suffer from PMS are themselves more likely to suffer. Personal attitudes to the naturalness of menstruation play a role in PMS. Negative attitudes to menstruation and the feminine role are more common in women who suffer from PMS than those who do not.

WHAT CAUSES PMS?

The answer is: we do not know. Virtually every system in the body has been implicated. It is known that the symptoms of PMS occur in the second half of the cycle after ovulation (the production of an egg). So it is assumed that there is some association between this and PMS. What this association is remains unknown.

The menstrual cycle is a highly complex and finely balanced series of events. It involves hormones, the central nervous system, psychological factors, basic cellular substances such as essential fatty acids and protoglandins, and diet. The relationships between all of these have not yet been established. One thing, however, is certain: there is no single cause for PMS, but some sort of imbalance between all systems in the body which still has to be sorted out.

WHAT ARE THE SYMPTOMS OF PMS?

More than 150 symptoms have been attributed to PMS. It is the timing of these, rather than the actual symptoms, that is important in diagnosing PMS. However, in managing PMS, the symptoms themselves are important, as each of these is treated differently. Many of these symptoms are identical to those of recognised medical and psychiatric disorders; they differ only in duration and in their predictable relationships to periods.

To simplify the many variations of symptoms, it is possible to group them into four main areas.

• Tension, irritability and anxiety. This is the most common group.

• Weight gain, abdominal bloating and tenderness, breast congestion and pain. Weight increase is usually around three pounds. With increasing age, this weight is not always lost completely after a period.

• Increased appetite and cravings, especially for chocolate and refined sugars. This indulgence usually occurs during stressful situations.

• Depression, withdrawal and suicidal ideas. Women complain of lethargy, confusion and difficulty in verbalising. These are the women who often consult a psychiatrist first.

While experiencing PMS, many women feel guilty about the way they are treating their partners and children. For example, a woman might lash out at her children, either verbally or physically, and will then get upset about her behaviour. Relationships with partners can also be put under strain at this time, which only adds to the problems. By the time a woman seeks help from her doctor, she has usually lost her self-esteem, sometimes even saying that she thinks she is going mad.

HOW DO I KNOW IF
I SUFFER FROM PMS?

One in four women who attend PMS clinics does not have PMS at all; instead, she is suffering from some other medical or psychiatric condition. For this reason, women should seek professional help in making a correct diagnosis. Once this has been done, a self-help programme can begin.

A woman who feels she may be suffering from PMS is advised to start a diary. Every night for three consecutive months, she writes down her main feelings and symptoms of the day, as well as what she has eaten and drunk – especially the amount of tea, coffee, chocolate, cakes and biscuits. Each symptom is given a score of severity from one to ten. These daily symptom ratings are the only means of diagnosing PMS. It is also helpful if a woman is able to involve her partner with the daily diary, since this will help him to understand the problem more fully.

It is interesting to note that while keeping the three-month diary, some women find that their PMS symptoms are not quite as severe. The symptoms may still be present, but the women have developed a greater insight and understanding, which is in itself a form of treatment.

WHAT SHOULD I DO IF
I THINK I HAVE PMS?

After keeping a diary for three months, the woman should then visit her doctor, remembering to bring her diary with her. This is extremely important, as a woman may have PMS along with some other disorder which could be medical, psychiatric or gynaecological. For example, a woman with heavy periods may be anaemic, which will make her feel much worse premenstrually. If she decides to treat her PMS on her own, it will not improve until her anaemia has been dealt with first.

The diagnosis of PMS should not be made without taking a full medical history and performing a clinical examination. The woman's social circumstances should also be assessed, along with her lifestyle and diet. It is only when all of these areas have been analysed that a suitable plan of action can be constructed.

WHAT IF MY DOCTOR IS
NOT SYMPATHETIC?

Most modern GPs are now well-versed in the problems surrounding PMS. Some, however, may not have a particular interest in this area, so it is advisable to attend someone who has.

Family planning clinics all have doctors who are experienced in dealing with PMS. When making an appointment, it is important to tell the receptionist the reason for your visit so that you are given enough time to discuss things. It is money well spent to get the correct diagnosis and to find a management scheme that suits your individual needs.

HOW CAN I HELP MYSELF?

Once you are diagnosed as having PMS, a great deal of help is within your own power. The way in which you may have to reorganise your life is a very personal thing; it should be seen as team-work involving your doctor, your partner and family, and yourself.

Make a list of the major problems that affect you while you are suffering from PMS, then organise ways in which to avoid them. Although this really works, it is this very type of self-focus that so many women deny themselves.

I am at home all day and cannot cope with the usual household chores before my period.

One of the most common symptoms of PMS is stress. We all experience stress in our lives and we usually cope. The secret of coping in the weeks before a period is organisation. Don't set deadlines for yourself during your premenstrual week. Arrange to do the things that you enjoy.

Get as much of the ironing done as you can during the first two weeks of your cycle; cook double amounts of meals and freeze them.

During the premenstrual stage of your cycle, get your hair done, meet a friend for lunch, go to a play. Learn relaxation techniques. Take long, warm baths and listen to your favourite music. Take the dog for a walk, do yoga, have a massage. Wear clothes in which you feel really comfortable.

I feel guilty about the way I treat my children in the week before my period. I lash out at them for no reason and am then filled with remorse.

This is a common problem which can also be helped by organisation. Get a friend to take the younger ones for a few hours in the morning (you can repay the favour when she needs your help). Get your partner to take the children out in the evening or at weekends and arrange for someone else to pick them up from school. Get your partner to supervise the homework. Organise clothes and lunches the previous night, then go to bed early and get up early so there is no morning panic. Have a 'Mum's week' once a month when other members of the family have to see to your needs for a change. By talking to the children (even the three- and four-year-olds) at their own levels, you will be surprised at what they are able to understand and that they would like to help in whatever ways they can. Another useful tip is to count to ten before you explode. It's much better than lashing out and feeling bad afterwards.

I treat my partner badly when I'm premenstrual.
It is helpful to involve your partner in keeping your diary. Communication is vital. He too may be suffering during this time, so be sure you talk to him – he can't be expected to know instinctively how you are feeling. This will also give him the opportunity to discuss the ways in which he can help with any lifestyle rearrangements.

I find it difficult to cope at work while I'm premenstrual.
There is no virtue in suffering by yourself – and in making others suffer too. Don't just grin and bear it – make out a coping strategy that suits you. Again, the secret of success is organisation. Make sure you get up in time so there's no last-minute rush. Try to look your best, but wear loose-fitting, comfortable clothes, with a bra one size larger than usual if you have breast symptoms.

Breakfast is a must – yoghurt, a slice of toast, a glass of orange juice with a spoonful of honey if you don't feel like eating. If driving to work causes stress, use public transport, walk, or arrange for a lift. If you have flexible hours, use these to your advantage.

Have a snack of fruit-and-nut bars for morning and afternoon breaks and treat yourself to a nice lunch. Then take a walk in the fresh air instead of sitting in a noisy canteen. Find a pleasant park or a church in which to sit and relax for fifteen minutes. Avoid junk foods as these will only make you feel worse. If possible, avoid important meetings until around the time your period has started. After work, go home to a warm bath, a good film and then early to bed – the dust can gather for another week.

WILL IT HELP IF I
CHANGE WHAT I EAT?

Yes, it certainly will. This is why it is important to document what you have consumed in your diary. When they are premenstrual, many women find that they increase their intake of coffee and refined sugars in cakes, biscuits and chocolates. It is only by writing things down that one becomes aware of this. When your blood sugar level drops, you feel awful; if this is added to PMS, you feel even worse. It is important to keep your blood sugar level up, but not by eating chocolates as this causes mood swings from high to low. Cravings for things like refined sugars are common during this time. Once you understand that this only makes things worse, you can persuade your body that it doesn't need that bar of chocolate. The secret is to eat good food, and to do so little and often. It may suit you better to have five small meals per day rather than three big ones.

Avoid junk foods and those which are high in salt, as these may contribute to excess swelling. If anxiety is part of your PMS problem, reduce your intake of coffee and tea. Try mineral water and herbal teas instead. If you have severe PMS, you should also avoid alcohol. Eat plenty of fruit and vegetables, especially if you are constipated.

Make any changes in your diet slowly. Be patient, and the results will be lasting. Sugar, salt and caffeine are the three main substances to avoid. If you need a sweetener, use honey. If you are overweight, it will be helpful to lose a few pounds. But don't start a diet when you are premenstrual – it only leads to disaster.

EXERCISE

Exercise is good for everyone, so it is good to try to increase your level of fitness. Whatever form of exercise you choose, it should be enjoyable for you. About twenty minutes per day is usually enough to improve muscle tone and general health.

Learn to relax, to communicate, to get a good night's sleep and to eat well. It takes time to get the balance right, as no single factor will help on its own. During the first few months of your self-help regime, be sure to keep your diary every night so your plans can be refined as required.

PMS AND ADOLESCENCE

Though PMS is not so common during the teenage years, when it does occur it only adds to the difficulties often associated with puberty. Adolescent PMS should be dealt with with sensitivity and understanding, as the condition can diminish school performance and can scar attitudes towards femininity and sexuality for life. Some teenage girls may be embarrassed about talking to the GP, so this should be done with care and patience. Dieting should be discouraged, with the channels of communication being kept open at all times.

Clumsiness is often a problem for premenstrual teenagers. It can lead to teasing at school which will in turn increase stress and make things worse. Like adult women, the adolescent should develop her own relaxation techniques and coping strategies. Acne can be another severe premenstrual problem; medication should be prescribed by the GP.

In spite of PMS, the teenager must learn that both homework and housework must be dealt with; letting either of these pile up will only lead to increased stress. Therefore a school project that is due during the premenstrual period should be tackled in the first half of the cycle.

PMS AND THE MENOPAUSE

As long as the ovaries are functioning, PMS can still occur. Around the start of the change of life, it is often difficult to decide whether one is suffering from the symptoms of the menopause or from PMS. PMS can worsen at this time, so the diagnosis is again extremely important. It may require a hormonal blood test to discover exactly what is going on.

MEDICAL TREATMENTS FOR PMS
AND THEIR SUCCESS RATES

With the causes of PMS remaining uncertain, and with a wide variety of treatment options available, a rational approach to this treatment is needed. Many women find that the self-help management methods are helpful and that nothing more is required. However, others may find that they need further help and will therefore opt for one of the many medical treatment options.

Two simple over-the-counter remedies worth mentioning are vitamin B_6 and oil of evening primrose. If you suffer mainly from depression and negative feelings before a period, vitamin B_6 (100mg daily) may be helpful. You may have to take it for about two months before you feel the effects, so be patient. As with many vitamins, it is harmful to take this one in excess.

If you have breast symptoms, oil of evening primrose capsules (four to eight per day) are effective and should be taken throughout the entire cycle. They are fairly expensive but provide excellent relief of breast discomfort and pain.

If this regime does not work, you will then have to proceed to stage two of the management programme which will involve the use of prescription drugs. Their use depends not only on the severity of the symptoms but also on the type of symptoms.

HORMONE THERAPY

Progesterone (one of the natural female hormones) is available in suppository, injection or tablet form. It is a particularly successful cycle regulator but is not a contraceptive. There are cheaper progestrogens (synthetic hormones) which can be taken during the second half of the cycle. These work occasionally but their use is limited. If contraception is also required, some relief may be obtained from the progesterone-only pill (the mini-pill).

In some studies, the oral contraceptive pill has been shown to decrease the incidence of PMS, and it also has the added advantage of providing effective contraception. It requires a trial period of two months to determine whether it is effective in any individual case and it is usually recommended that it be taken with vitamin B_6.

When premenstrual pain is a problem, substances called prostaglandin synthetase inhibitors are useful. These should be taken three times a day from the onset of pain until the second or third day of the period. Women with ulcers should not take these tablets.

Water pills or diuretics are occasionally used when weight gain and fluid retention are major problems. Another drug, Spironolactone, is sometimes used, but its use must be carefully monitored.

Bromocriptine is a drug that is useful for breast symptoms if oil of evening primrose has proved unsuccessful. It has nasty side-effects, however, and requires careful monitoring, and it is used only in very specific cases.

Some women respond well to behavioural therapy and psychotherapy, particularly if the major symptoms are depression or aggression.

By careful management through stages one and two, most women will respond positively and will be able to resume normal living. It must be stated that some treatments may last for only a year or two, after which PMS may return. If this happens, it is usually 'back to the drawing board', starting again with the diary and a visit to the doctor.

FINAL CHOICES

For a few women, more drastic measures are required, bringing them to stage three. The object here is to stop the ovaries from functioning altogether by interfering with hormone levels. This is done with drugs such as Danazol, gonadotrophin releasing hormone analogues and oestradiol implants. All may have serious side-effects and are used only under the supervision of a specialist.

The final choice is to have surgery involving a hysterectomy and the removal of both ovaries. This is a drastic step and is usually only performed because of severe premenstrual violence. It is the definitive cure, but at a huge cost. The woman then requires hormone replacement therapy (HRT) which, according to recent research, can itself cause PMS-type symptoms.

PMS is debilitating for both women and their families. In the last fifteen years, it has become more widely recognised and accepted by the medical profession as a serious problem.

Many women who seek help have already lost their self-esteem and self-confidence, and need to adopt a positive approach. Education of family and friends and a better understanding of the problem are steps towards alleviating much of the suffering this condition causes.

It is up to every woman to take charge of her own life, not to suffer in silence as so many of our ancestors did. This can be done very successfully with a little help from your family doctor.

Dr Valerie Donnelly MB, BCh, LRCP and SI, MRCOG is a Research Fellow and Clinical Tutor in University College, Dublin, and a Registrar in Obstetrics and Gynaecology at the National Maternity Hospital, Holles Street, Dublin.

SEXUAL DIFFICULTIES

MARY O'CONOR

It is probably not quite true to say that there was no sex in Ireland before The Late Late Show, *but there was certainly no such thing as sex therapy. If anyone was bold enough to be enjoying sex, they couldn't have admitted it. On the other side of the coin, nobody could admit that they were having sexual difficulties. There must surely have been a lot of misery and frustration behind closed bedroom doors.*

Today, trained sex therapists like Mary O'Conor are there to help those who are having problems to experience, perhaps for the first time, the joy of sex . . .

SEX AND SEXUALITY

Sex – the word guaranteed to sell magazines and newspapers, attract viewers to film and television programmes, rouse the 'high moral ground' groups to action and generate many hours of discussion. Sex is what everybody thinks everybody else is having a much better time doing, despite the fact that almost everybody encounters problems at some stage in their lives. Sex is something that affects us all in one way or another. It is also one of the few things that doesn't cost any money, can be a lot of fun and enriches relationships.

Sex affects us from the moment of birth. The very first words used to describe us are 'It's a boy' or 'It's a girl'. We are then assigned either blue or pink. At a very early age we start to pick up messages about what our parents and society in general expect of the little blue or pink bundle. 'What a pretty dress!' or 'Have you lots of dolls?' as opposed to 'Big boys don't cry!', 'What team do you support?'

As we develop sexually, we get many mixed messages about sex. The message from parents is usually not to do it at all. From the school, we get some information about the 'nuts and bolts', together with the Church's teaching, and some contraceptive information as well. At the same time, the message from our peers is that boys should be trying to get it as often as possible with as many as possible, and that girls shouldn't give it unless they want to be labelled 'fast'. Meanwhile, films, television and novels are leading us to believe that everybody is at it all the time, with either their own or somebody else's partner; bodies are perfect with not a spot or stretchmark or extra flab in sight; everybody is ready, willing and able to do it at any time, and is probably simultaneously or multi-orgasmic. Is it any wonder, then, that people often feel sexually inadequate and start to encounter problems. This does not even account for specific traumas like rape or incest which in themselves would have negative effects on sexuality.

Guilt is a subject that people talk about a lot in reference to sexuality, and this is easy to understand. If a child remembers that his or her questions about sex were not answered, that the television was turned off whenever anything vaguely sexual came on (or parents hiding uncomfortably behind newspapers) and sex being generally a taboo subject, then they are quite likely to feel guilty when they get to the stage of actually enjoying it. Nobody said anything about enjoying it! If it was never spoken of and if people were uncomfortable with it, then it must be wrong. There is also the guilt attached to discovering our own bodies as children. We are actively discouraged ('Take that hand away') and are often told that nudity is to be avoided at all costs. It is not very surprising, then, that so many people end up ashamed of their own bodies and uncomfortable with nudity. While certainly not advocating that we go around without clothes (with our climate it would be ridiculous), we can still learn a lot from our children who somehow instinctively know when it is no longer appropriate to be undressed in front of others. This happens around the same time as they begin knocking before entering their parents' bedroom – and when they rightly expect the same treatment from their parents.

Masturbation is another area about which there is tremendous guilt, but it is after all the best way to learn about our sexual responses. How can we tell a partner what we like if we don't know ourselves? Masturbation helps to increase awareness of our own body responses. For those temporarily or permanently without a partner, it provides a relief of tension. It can help men to develop ejaculatory control. And it does not make you blind.

We get our information about sex from a variety of sources – a bit from friends, a bit from siblings, a bit from books, magazines and videos. The trouble is that sometimes we put the bits together wrongly and give ourselves unnecessary worry. The schools have made great advances with their sex education programmes, but these would be even more effective if parents were also involved. If the parents knew exactly what was being taught at school, they could then undertake to put the human side on it. Sex can happen between two consenting adults who scarcely know each other, but if it can be conveyed to children how much better it is in the context of a loving relationship, then that message should stay with them. Parents are role models, whether they like it or not and whether the children like it or not. If they can be role models

221

of a good relationship – which therefore implies a good sexual one – so much the better. Also, the more comfortable the child will be and the easier he or she will be in asking questions.

Asking questions raises the question of abuse. Many years ago, a colleague told me that she had noticed that she was getting very little response from clients to her question about whether there had been any abuse or incest in the family. She decided to change the way she put the question, asking if the person had ever been touched in any way that made them feel uncomfortable, or if they had been shown any pictures or told any stories of a sexual nature that made them feel uneasy. She suddenly found that she was getting a greater response as people told stories of various incidents they remembered. These incidents had bothered them, but they didn't feel they were as serious as the abuse stories that made the headlines.

Abuse and incest are now spoken of more often, but for many people, abuse and incest mean penetrative intercourse by either a father or a close family member. However, sex therapists encounter people who have a sexual problem resulting from abuse that is not necessarily penetrative sex. What may seem trivial to one person may have been enough to cause a major problem in later life to another and it is important to bear this in mind.

SEXUAL PROBLEMS

Most people experience sexual difficulties at some time in their lives, and that is perfectly normal. There can be many reasons for this, for example, a new baby, pressure at work, tiredness from work or the children, living with the in-laws etc. These problems usually need only time to resolve themselves. However, when a sexual problem is there for more than six months, and when physical causes have been ruled out by checking with your doctor, it is time to seek help. In the old days, people often consulted a priest initially, but now it is often the GP or gynaecologist to whom they turn. However, many people are too embarrassed to go to their doctor, so they go directly to a sex therapist. We are used to people being shy and embarrassed when they first come to us and we try very hard to put them at their ease. For most people, it is the first time that they have ever admitted to anybody except their partner that there is a problem and so it is a big hurdle to be jumped. Clients often talk about having had the telephone number for ages but being too nervous to make the call. They eventually feel there was a load lifted from their shoulders when they finally come to see us.

FEMALE SEXUAL PROBLEMS

Vaginismus

This is a condition that affects a surprisingly large number of women. The muscles at the entrance to the vagina tighten so completely that the woman is unable to allow penetration of any sort, even a tampon during a period. She also cannot allow a full gynaecological examination. Women with vaginismus speak of feelings of isolation, of not being a complete woman. They would often look around a crowded room and feel that they were the only one with this problem. They usually feel they are beyond help, so they are surprised to hear that the success rate in the treatment of vaginismus is high.

Dyspareunia

In this case, the woman can actually allow penetration by the penis but to do so causes severe pain. So naturally enough, she does not look forward to intercourse one little bit. A medical examination is always necessary to rule out any physical reason for the pain before treatment would be considered by the therapist.

Orgasmic difficulties

A woman may feel she is missing out if she thinks she is not reaching orgasm. Sometimes it is her partner who feels he is not 'good enough' if she is not experiencing orgasms. A sex therapy view is that we are all ultimately responsible for our own orgasm. If we want to learn more about our own body's responses, it is entirely appropriate to seek help. A word here about simultaneous orgasm or 'coming together'. Quite often, couples

223

would state this as one of their goals for treatment. To my mind, it is an unrealistic expectation. When you consider that the average orgasm lasts between ten and twenty seconds, and that an average sexual encounter takes between fifteen and twenty minutes, the probability of both people hitting that particular twenty seconds together is extremely remote. Nice if it happens but very unlikely!

MALE SEXUAL PROBLEMS

Erectile difficulties

Men often have anxieties about erections and all men experience difficulties at some stage in their lives. What is called performance anxiety ('Will I get it up, and if I do, will it stay up?') happens to most men at some stage, but it may only take a few unsuccessful experiences for it to become a problem. When I ask people who are having erection problems if they honestly believe that they are never again going to get an erection, they tell me not to be ridiculous. Erectile difficulties respond very well to sex therapy although it would be necessary to be checked out medically first, particularly if there are no erections at all. (Medical treatment for impotence is discussed in the chapter, 'Men's Problems'.)

Premature ejaculation

This occurs when the man ejaculates too quickly and sex is not satisfactory for one or both partners. Generally speaking, a woman takes longer to get aroused than a man (although not usually in masturbation). If he comes too soon and she is only getting there, and this happens regularly, then something needs to change. Premature ejaculation responds well to therapy.

Retarded ejaculation

This is the opposite situation. It occurs when the man cannot ejaculate at all, or when it takes so long for him to reach this point that it is unsatisfactory for one or both partners. This is not as common a complaint as premature ejaculation, but it can also be treated in therapy.

Lack of desire

A problem common to both sexes is lack of desire – 'gone off it' or, in some cases, 'never on it'. Everybody goes through stages in their lives when sex is the last thing on their mind, and that is understandable. But if the lack of desire lasts for an unacceptably long period, then help should be sought. Quite often, one partner has a much stronger sex drive than the other, and this is when there must be compromise. For instance, if she wants sex at least four times a week and he is happy with just once, then there has to be negotiation. Couples find that if they have established ground rules for themselves (in this case maybe twice a week but with a real effort on both parts to make it special in some way), there is far less friction. Couples with this lack of desire usually find that the sex therapy programme helps them to make a fresh start sexually and to think about sex in a different way.

As we are living for far longer than people used to, we are often faced with having sex with the same person for thirty or forty years. Therefore we really do need to put a little effort into bringing variety into our sex lives. Otherwise we will get bored no matter how much we love our partner. Nobody wants their favourite food every time they eat. Likewise with sex. So think about variety. A different place. A different time. Clothes on instead of off. Different lighting. Surprise your partner. Take a bath or shower together. Give each other a massage with an agreement to go no further. Read a book like Alex Comfort's *The Joy of Sex*. Let your imagination go. It can be great fun – and it's free!

TREATMENT

Sex therapy can help by changing one or both partners' attitude to sex, by helping to increase understanding of our own and our partner's needs, and by teaching techniques that will help overcome particular problems. For people to seek treatment, they need first to acknowledge to each other that a problem exists. They have to talk about it. Sometimes this can be difficult if people are very shy, or if one person is afraid of offending the other. A possible way out of this is to look at one of the Lover's

Guide videos that are available at video stores. While the bodies we see in these videos are usually far too perfect to bear any comparison to the great majority of us, the videos are good starting points for talking. If a video is not possible, then perhaps reading a piece from a problem page in a magazine, or referring to an appropriate radio item will help to get the ball rolling. You can be pretty sure that if you are worried about a particular problem, then your partner probably is also, and would welcome the chance to talk it through.

When a couple goes to a therapist, they have an initial session together during which the therapist explores the problem with them and tells them what sex therapy involves. This is followed by a detailed history-taking of both partners which is done individually and is the only time the couple are seen separately. The history-taking explores their family backgrounds, how their parents related to each other, how they related to their parents and siblings, their sex education, early sexual experiences, and personal and sexual development. It also goes in depth into their perception of themselves and of their partner. The therapist will want to make sure that the couple does not also have a relationship problem. If this is the case, counselling will be suggested before the sexual problem is tackled.

By the time the history-making is completed, the therapist knows a lot about the clients and their problem. They too have become at ease when talking with the therapist. This relationship is important as people really do need to trust the therapist if treatment is to succeed.

When they are seen together again, the therapist relates what he or she has learned about the couple and the possible origins of their problem. The couple should then have a fairly good understanding of what has happened to them previously, and the circumstances that have brought about the current situation. Then treatment begins.

Sex therapy differs from relationship counselling in that therapy is very much behaviour-oriented. Right from the beginning, the couple are given specific tasks to accomplish which are normally called 'homework'. Discussion about how they got on with the homework, and instructions for the following week, take up much of the time during subsequent visits with the therapist. Quite often, a change takes place in the relationship as couples find they become much closer now that they are able to talk freely about their problem. As they experience changes in attitude, and see physical results which prove that things are changing, it gets very exciting for them.

Therapy is seen as a chance to begin again, going right back to the courtship stage. For the first few weeks there is a ban on intercourse so that the couple can fully explore and enjoy each other's bodies without the pressure to perform.

Apart from seeing couples, sex therapists will also see single clients – those who have no partner, or whose partner for some reason or another cannot or will not attend. Although it ultimately takes two to tango, a lot of very useful work can be done with single clients, so they should not be afraid to seek help.

A topic that is bound up with our sexuality and that we need to think about is hygiene. When somebody starts sex therapy, they are given three one-hour homework sessions a week which have to start with either a bath or shower. There is a good reason for this. When we first start dating, we take tremendous care with our appearance, but perhaps we could all be guilty of taking our partners for granted as time goes by and not taking as much care as we should. There is the nice feeling of comfort when one is in a long-term relationship, but do we let our standards slip at the same time? How big a turn-on are greasy hair, stubble, bad breath, monthly baths or strong body odour? Even without any added extras like deodorant, one of the nicest things is the natural perfume of a freshly cleansed body and newly washed hair.

They undertake to do homework which involves massage and becoming totally familiar with one's own body. We call these massage exercises 'sensate focus' because the focus is on the sensual rather than the sexual. The aim is to reduce anxiety about sexual performance and instead to increase awareness of how to give and receive pleasure. Gradually, more steps are added which are tailored to meet the particular problem. As well as the

homework, there are information-giving sessions with the
therapist and relaxation exercises, all of which help. Therapy
takes between ten and twenty weeks. Clients are usually seen on
a weekly basis. There is a lot of fun involved as people either
discover or rediscover the joy of sex. Clients find that they are
looking forward to their time together and ultimately to having a
more satisfying sex life. No treatment can guarantee complete
success, but sex therapy does have quite high success rates.
There are many satisfied clients but we do not get any referrals
from them, as nobody tells anybody else they have been in
therapy.

WHERE TO GO FOR HELP

Quite often, the first person who is approached about sexual
problems is the family doctor. If that is not comfortable for you,
any of the recognised counselling services or family planning
clinics will be able to advise you. Be aware that anybody can
call themselves a therapist, so ask about qualifications and training.
The British Association of Sexual and Marital Therapists has
accredited certain courses and they have members in this
country. Don't be afraid to go to a therapist if you have a
problem that is not mentioned here. I have listed the most
common problems, but there are many others. You can certainly
benefit from talking with somebody who will help you decide if
treatment is appropriate. And if you have been putting off doing
something about it, give yourself a little push. Help is available –
it's up to you.

Mary O'Conor is a qualified sex therapist and relationship
counsellor in private practice at the Baggot Clinic, 32 Upper
Baggot Street, Dublin 4. She is a member of the British
Association for Sexual and Marital Therapy and of the Irish
Association for Counselling.

SEXUALLY TRANSMITTED DISEASES

DR FIONA MULCAHY

Sexually transmitted diseases (STDs), also known as venereal diseases, are among the most commonly acquired infections. Anyone who is involved in unprotected, casual sex runs the risk of becoming infected. Men and women from all social classes, religions and nationalities get STDs. By their very nature, these diseases involve secrecy, guilt and embarrassment.

The most frightening sexually transmitted disease is AIDS. But there are many other STDs and these too are on the increase. As symptoms may not appear until the disease is well advanced, Dr Fiona Mulcahy, Consultant in Genito-urinary Medicine, advises anyone who has had a sexual encounter that may have put them at risk of infection to see their doctor immediately . . .

WHAT ARE STDS?

Many sexually transmitted diseases (STDs) have no symptoms, but some may cause unpleasant and sometimes harmful effects. The majority can be cured when treated appropriately. It is now thought that the HIV virus which causes AIDS can be more easily passed on if one sexual partner already has another sexually transmitted disease.

If you suspect you have put yourself at risk of picking up an infection, you should be diagnosed and treated as early as possible. Preferably, this should be at a clinic specialising in STDs where appropriate tests can be carried out by doctors who are trained in this area of medicine.

It is important to remember that STDs are not transmitted by sharing cutlery or crockery, in swimming pools, from toilet seats, or by non-sexual contact with infected people. STDs are caused by bacteria, viruses and other microscopic organisms which are present in the blood, semen, body fluids, or the pubic area of an infected person.

GONORRHOEA

Gonorrhoea is caused by bacteria. It can affect the vagina, the cervix (the lower part of the womb), the urethra (the pipe that carries urine from the bladder), the rectum (back passage), even the throat. The disease is passed on through vaginal sex (when the man puts his penis into the woman's vagina), anal sex (the penis is put into the rectum) or oral sex (when partners lick or suck each other's sexual parts). It may be possible to pass gonorrhoea from mouth to mouth with very deep french kissing, but this is rare. The bacteria cannot live outside the body, so it cannot be passed on from toilet seats, swimming pools or by sharing cups and towels.

Most women who get gonorrhoea do not notice anything unusual until the infection has spread from the cervix. Some may then notice an unusual change in the natural discharge of the vagina which may be yellow or greenish in colour. They may also experience some pain on passing urine, and occasionally a sore throat.

Men will notice a white, yellow or green fluid coming from the tip of the penis which may stain the underpants.

Gonorrhoea has a short incubation period and the symptoms appear within a week or two after exposure. Treatment is essential. Although some of the discharges or other symptoms may clear up by themselves, gonorrhoea may still be present and can go on to cause chronic problems and damage. In men, untreated gonorrhoea can lead to inflammation of the testes and the prostate gland.

In women, untreated gonorrhoea can lead to severe pelvic inflammatory disease. This is an inflammation of the fallopian tubes which can cause infertility or ectopic pregnancy (a life-threatening condition in which the pregnancy is located in the fallopian tubes). A pregnant woman could then pass the infection on to her newborn baby, causing an eye infection (gonoccocal conjunctivitis) which can lead to blindness.

Diagnosis and treatment
Gonorrhoea is diagnosed by special tests which involve taking specific swabs from the urethra and cervix in women and from the penis in men.

Treatment is both easy and effective. It usually involves a penicillin-type antibiotic, although some types of gonorrhoea infections are resistant to penicillin and thus require other antibiotics.

It is common to pick up more than one type of sexual infection at the same time. Therefore, after the gonorrhoea has been cleared, other infections may come to light which will also need treatment.

CHLAMYDIA TRACHOMATIS
Chlamydia trachomatis is a small organism which, like gonorrhoea, may affect the urethra, cervix, anus and throat. Although it shares many of the signs and symptoms associated with gonorrhoea, it can lie dormant for much longer.

This infection can have devastating effects on women, as it

may remain silent for many years before it presents with late complications. *Chlamydia* infection is thought to be one of the most common causes today of pelvic inflammatory disease and infertility in sexually-active women. Women who have *chlamydia* at the time of childbirth may pass the infection on to their babies. This causes a severe eye infection (*Chlamydia opthalmia neonatorum*) or an infection of the ears and lungs.

Men who are suffering from *chlamydia* will usually notice a discharge or fluid coming from the tip of the penis. Unlike gonorrhoea, however, this discharge is clearer and may be mistaken for dribbling which occurs after passing urine.

Diagnosis and treatment
Chlamydia is diagnosed by swabs which are sent to a laboratory for identification of the micro-organism. Once it has been diagnosed, its treatment is simple and involves a two-week course of antibiotics.

HERPES SIMPLEX VIRUS

There are two types of *Herpes simplex* virus, types I and II. These viruses are almost identical and can only be differentiated in the laboratory. Traditionally, *Herpes simplex* type I was thought to cause only cold sores on the mouth and around the nose. *Herpes simplex II* was thought to cause the genital-type herpes infection. However, it is now known that both types can be found in both areas.

Herpes simplex is passed on through sexual contact from one genital area to another. It can also be passed from the mouth where there is a cold sore to the genital area during oral sex. *Herpes simplex* can sometimes affect a finger, causing a herpetic whitlow (a painful cluster of blisters) which may also be a source of infection.

It is important to remember that *Herpes simplex* is highly contagious. The greatest risk is in the first forty-eight hours of an active infection. The incubation period is about a week.

Genital herpes in females may cause a number of symptoms.

232

There may be stinging and itching in the genital area for twenty-four hours prior to the development of other signs. The woman may feel generally unwell, with some aches and pains in the genital area which may spread down the legs. Twenty-four to forty-eight hours later, small blisters may develop along the vulva. Blisters that are visible on the outside may also be an indication that there are more blisters inside the vagina, the cervix and rectum.

In men, small blisters develop underneath the foreskin or around the head of the penis. When these blisters burst, they form small ulcers which are extremely painful to the touch, particularly if they come in contact with urine. The pain may be so severe that it is impossible to pass urine.

The main complication with genital herpes is that about half of those who contract it will suffer recurrent attacks. Generally, however, recurrences are less severe than the original attack. To limit further attacks, it is important to avoid trigger factors. Stress is one of the major factors, so avoiding any physical or emotional stress is important.

Diagnosis and treatment

Diagnosis is made by the doctor on examination and can be confirmed with swabs sent for culture of the virus. This takes approximately two weeks, but treatment should be started immediately.

In the first acute attack, treatment is with anti-viral tablets Acyclovir (Zovirax). They help to decrease the length of time the attack is present and improve the symptoms dramatically. Other measures that decrease the pain include salt baths (at least three or four times a day), cold showers and pain-killers. If there is difficulty in passing urine, it may help to try urinating in a warm bath. In rare cases, the patient may have to be admitted to hospital for treatment.

Women who have had a history of *Herpes simplex* genital infection are strongly advised to inform their obstetrician when they become pregnant. If there is a fresh infection at the time of delivery, the baby may have to be delivered by Caesarian section. This is necessary to prevent the transmission of the infection to the baby, which can cause severe complications such as meningitis, even death in some cases.

GENITAL WARTS

Genital warts are becoming increasingly common in both men and women. They are caused by a virus infection called the *Human papilloma* virus which is transmitted by sexual contact with an infected person. The warm areas around the genitals are ideal places for the growth of this virus. It may take between three weeks and a year for genital warts to develop after you have first been infected. They appear as small fleshy lumps which may become larger and which are commonly grouped together. Sometimes, the warts are very small and flat and may be hidden in areas such as the anus and vagina.

In women, the warts are found mainly on the vulva, but they may also be detected in the vagina and around the cervix. In men, they are found underneath the foreskin and on the head of the penis. They are sometimes found down the urethra (the pipe in the penis) and are therefore not always visible.

Both men and women may also get warts around the anus. When these are detected, they should be treated as quickly as possible, as they may become much larger and more difficult to remove as time goes on.

There is some evidence to suggest that warts are linked to cancer of the cervix in women, and cancer of the anus in men. It is strongly recommended that women who have had genital warts, or whose partners have had them, have a cervical smear test once a year.

Treatment

Treatment for genital warts is usually given over a number of weeks. It includes the use of podophyllum lotion and trichloroacetic acid, a strong acid that is applied by a doctor or nurse. Cryotherapy, which involves freezing the warts, may also be used. Larger warts may be removed surgically, under either a local or a general anaesthetic. Sexual contact should be avoided until the warts have been eradicated. A condom should then be used for up to three months after clearance. Partners should also be investigated and checked for warts, as it is probable that they will recur if one partner remains infected.

TRICHOMONIASIS

Trichomoniasis is an infection caused by a tiny parasite which may infect the vagina or the urethra. It is asymptomatic (causes no symptoms) in men, who may not be aware that they are carrying this infection. When a woman comes in contact with it, she may develop symptoms within a few days to three weeks.

In women, trichomoniasis causes a yellow-greenish frothy discharge which has a fishy odour. It may also cause a burning sensation in the vagina and around the vulva, with staining of the underwear. Unlike other infections, however, it causes no major complications.

Treatment

Treatment consists of a course of antibiotics which will effectively cure the infection. Since this infection lies dormant in males, it is essential that partners are treated with a similar course of antibiotics.

THRUSH (CANDIDIASIS)

Thrush is caused by a small organism that normally lives in the gut, in the mouth and on the skin. This organism is mainly *Candida albicans*, although other similar types of *candida* species are also present. In normal circumstances, *candida* is present and remains at a steady level in the body. Sometimes, however, this can multiply and cause discomfort. Since *candida* is a normal passenger in the body, it cannot be eradicated completely. Its multiplication is more likely to happen during pregnancy, in diabetics, in people who are taking antibiotics, or as a result of wearing tight-fitting nylon clothes. This can also occur through sexual contact with someone whose own levels of *candida* have also increased.

In women, candida causes itching and a vaginal discharge which is white and looks like cottage cheese. There may also be a swelling of the vulva, with some discomfort and pain in passing urine.

In men, the foreskin may be red and itchy; it may also split and become sore. There may also be a rash around the groin and in the creases around the testes and buttocks.

Diagnosis and treatment

Candidiasis may be diagnosed by taking a specific swab which counts the number of *candida* colonies present on the swab.

Treatment is usually straightforward and involves a cream for the skin and pessaries for the vagina. It is important for all partners to be treated as well, as they may be a source of re-infection.

HEPATITIS B

Hepatitis B is an infectious and potentially life-threatening infection caused by the Hepatitis B virus (HBV). It can occur in all body fluids, especially the blood. In western Europe, it is spread mainly by one of the following activities: having sex with an infected person; sharing needles with an infected person; or coming in contact with infectious body fluids (blood, saliva) found on needles or other sharp instruments. In other parts of the world, this virus is commonly spread from an infected mother to her unborn baby, and between close family contacts. The Hepatitis B virus is a hundred times more infectious than HIV and kills more people worldwide every year than AIDS.

HBV infects the liver. It may cause tiredness, muscle pain and weakness, and often jaundice (a yellowish colour to the skin and whites of the eyes). Symptoms of an acute infection may take six months to develop, resulting in death in approximately one case per 500. Clearance of the virus can take six months. About 10 per cent of cases remain carriers of the virus and are therefore infectious. These people also develop chronic liver disease, including cirrhosis and liver cancer, with an associated high death rate.

Diagnosis and treatment

HBV can be diagnosed by a special blood test. Although there is no effective treatment for an acute infection, new treatment possibilities exist for chronic carriers using the drug Interferon. However, HBV is preventable with the use of Hepatitis B vaccine. While vaccination prevents infection, it does not cure those who are already infected.

HIV AND AIDS

Human immunodeficiency virus (HIV) affects a person's immune system, rendering it susceptible to many infections, particularly other viruses, parasites and fungi. It is detectable in all body fluids, especially semen and blood. In Ireland, it is spread mainly by unprotected sex or by sharing needles with an infected person. Infected mothers can also pass the virus to their children *in utero* (during pregnancy), at delivery and during breast feeding. HIV is not spread by sharing cutlery, living accommodation, from toilet seats, swimming pools, shaking hands, hugging etc.

A person infected with HIV (HIV positive) will develop antibodies to the virus which are detectable in a blood test within three months of acquiring the infection. The individual will usually remain well for five to eight years before developing any symptoms of the virus. They are infectious during this time, however.

Early symptoms of HIV infection can be similar to glandular fever or flu. They include sore throat, swollen glands, fever, pains in the joints, skin rashes, and a general feeling of being unwell.

Acquired immune deficiency syndrome (AIDS) is not a disease in its own right. It occurs as the final stage of HIV infection because the body's immune defences have broken down and other diseases can then easily attack and become established. These include cancers, pneumonia, severe thrush and a wide range of other infections. Symptoms associated with later stages of the disease include significant weight loss, prolonged diarrhoea, chronic fungal infections of the skin and mouth, and symptoms specifically related to chest and brain infections. AIDS was originally known as 'Slim's Disease' because of the severe weight loss that comes with its later stages.

The pattern of the disease is such that patients will get very sick, then get better, then become sick again and so on over a period of years before they finally get an infection or tumour that does not respond to treatment.

Treatment

Major advances have been made in recent years in the treatment of these infections. Patients with AIDS may live for a number of years with a reasonable quality of life. Close monitoring of the immune system, with regular medical examinations and blood tests, will detect those who are most at risk of becoming ill. They may then be put on medications to improve their immune responses.

As sexually transmitted diseases become more common, it is vital for people to take greater responsibility for their health. Clearly the use of condoms will reduce the risk of acquiring an STD. However, when someone has exposed themselves to the possibility of acquiring a sexual infection, they must get medical advice immediately so that treatment can begin and their future sexual partners be protected.

Dr Fiona Mulcahy MD, FRCPI is a Consultant in Genito-urinary Medicine at St James's Hospital, Dublin, and she lectures in Trinity College, Dublin.

SKIN DISORDERS

DR SARAH ROGERS

The skin is the largest organ of the body. The average adult has two square yards of it, and it makes up about 15 per cent of your total weight.

Because skin is on the outside, where it can be seen, skin problems can not only make you feel unwell – they can also be very disfiguring and embarrassing. Someone with psoriasis or eczema may become extremely self-conscious about their appearance. A teenager may feel their life is in ruins because of a few spots. Fortunately there is a great deal that can be done today to help those suffering from skin conditions, as consultant dermatologist Dr Sarah Rogers explains.

THE WORK OF THE SKIN

The primary object of the skin is to give protection. It waterproofs us and keeps out harmful bacteria. Together with the lining of the nasal passages and tonsils, it is the first line in the body's defence against infection. The skin also plays a major role in the control of body temperature. When the skin is affected by a generalised, inflammatory disease such as severe eczema or psoriasis, it radiates heat. Sweating cools us down, so if children cannot sweat because of the absence of sweat glands, they are unable to lower their body temperature when they get infections, and as a consequence develop febrile convulsions.

The skin helps to regulate fluid balance. Excess sweating causes dehydration unless we drink plenty of fluids. Skin also protects us from the harmful effects of ultraviolet (UV) radiation by producing a pigment called melanin in response to UV rays. Mediterranean, Indian and black races are all well equipped to produce an even layer of melanin. Celtic skin, which accounts for 70 per cent of the Irish population, does not have this ability. People with such skin tend to freckle and burn and are more prone to skin cancer.

Lastly, but very importantly, the skin is a means of communication. It helps us to look attractive, can tell our age, our social background and even our occupation. In the Victorian era, it was important to have a white skin to show you were from the upper social classes; only peasants got brown in the sun. In this age of package holidays, being tanned indicates that you can afford to fly to the sun. It is also interpreted as denoting health which, of course, is not true.

Also not true are the old chestnuts that diet, allergy and stress play a major role in skin disease and that most skin conditions are infectious and contagious.

ACNE VULGARIS

Acne starts at puberty, occurs equally in both sexes and tends to get better by the late teens or twenties. It may first appear in women at a later age, even in their thirties. Acne occurs in at least 95 per cent of the population. In most people, it is mild and regarded as part of growing up. But that is not how the sufferer sees it. Acne causes much misery, since it strikes at an age when looking good is all-important. It may be quite a nasty disease in some, causing a great deal of discomfort and scarring.

In spite of what your mother may have told you, acne has absolutely nothing to do with diet or dirt. No amount of scrubbing will 'out these damned spots', nor will drinking copious amounts of water. Eating chips and hamburgers till they come out of your ears will not make acne worse – grease from the diet does not appear in the skin. Skin grease (sebum) is under hormonal control and is produced by the grease glands in response to testosterone (male hormone). Females have a small amount of testosterone, and therefore get acne just as males do. The spots are most numerous at the site of grease glands and so occur mainly on the face, shoulders and upper chest, although they may sometimes be more extensive. The classical acne rash consists of red spots (papules), pustules (yellow spots) and comedones (blackheads). If the individual spots are large, they are called nodules or cysts. These cause scarring.

Squeezing spots is an inevitable part of having acne. Put any acne sufferer in front of the mirror in a good light and they will squeeze, in spite of what their mothers and doctors advise them. In general, it does not do much harm. There are some young ladies who make a habit of picking the top off the spots before they have a chance to heal, leading to shallow white scarring. This is known as acne excoriée. Perhaps, rather than poking out blackheads, it is better to use a blackhead extractor which may be purchased from your local chemist.

Treatment

Anyone who reads magazines, watches TV and visits the local pharmacist will know that there is a whole range of treatments for acne. Those that can be purchased over the counter are often least effective and certainly will not clear severe acne. They dry the skin and make it peel and have a weak antibacterial effect. A common example is benzoyl peroxide (Panoxyl, Topex, Quinoderm). Sulphur has lost popularity because of its pungent smell and grittiness.

A visit to the doctor is necessary for many acne sufferers. Antibiotics are the mainstay of acne treatment. Some modern antibiotics can be applied to the skin in roll-on form and are effective for mild to moderate acne. For more severe forms, or for extensive disease, antibiotics are given as tablets. A course of topical antibiotic is three months, while a course of tablets is six months. Relapses after antibiotics are not uncommon and repeated courses may be necessary during the teenage years. Antibiotics cause very few side-effects other than, occasionally, vaginal thrush in women. Allergy to antibiotics for acne is rare. Long-term antibiotic treatment does not weaken the person's constitution or resistance to infection, though many parents frequently worry about this.

Oestrogen is good for treating acne since it counteracts the effects of testosterone or androgen. But the idea that the oral contraceptive pill (OCP) is good for acne is no longer true, as modern OCPs are low in oestrogen (female hormone). A pill called Dianette, which contains the anti-androgen cyproterone acetate, is the one OCP that is effective. It is particularly useful for women who want to take a contraceptive pill and have their acne treated at the same time. It is also given where antibiotics have failed to work. A minimum course lasts six months, but it may be given over a longer period.

For severe acne, the drug of choice is the vitamin A derivative, isotretinoin (Roaccutane). This drug has been revolutionary in the treatment of severe acne and is virtually 100 per cent effective. There is a very low relapse rate afterwards. It is an expensive and fairly toxic drug but it must be remembered that the toxicity is only for the duration of the course, which is from four to six months. The toxicity reverses when the drug is stopped. The only form of toxicity that does not reverse is that of damage to a developing baby (foetus). Because of its vitamin A-like actions, isotretinoin dries the skin and lips and may also cause aches and pains in muscles. It may cause blood cholesterol to rise and may cause disturbance of liver function. Throughout treatment, these conditions are carefully monitored by blood tests. For females of child-bearing age who take this drug, an

OCP is given at the same time because of the drug's tendency to damage the foetus. Roaccutane should be used only under the supervision of a consultant dermatologist.

The message for acne sufferers is that nowadays no one needs to go through years of misery with this disease. There is always a cure for any grade of acne, though it may take some months to reach the correct treatment.

ECZEMA/DERMATITIS

People often confuse these two terms but they mean the same thing. The term dermatitis tends to be reserved for contact dermatitis which is caused by something noxious touching the skin. An example is occupational dermatitis. Eczema affects somewhere between 15 and 25 per cent of the population at sometime in their lives.

A common form of eczema is seborrhoeic eczema. This is a dandruffy eczema which affects the scalp, eyebrows, sides of nose, front of chest and sometimes the back. It may also occur in crease areas under the arms and in the groins. A yeast organism, P. ovale, grows on the skin in seborrhoeic eczema. By using an anti-yeast agent, ketoconazole (Nizoral), in shampoo and/or cream form, this type of eczema is now totally controllable, if not curable. A prescription is required for Nizoral products.

The most common form of eczema is the one that starts in young children and is called infantile eczema. Its proper name is atopic eczema. It is inherited and is associated with asthma and hay fever. It can be made worse by proteins which are either inhaled (pollens, house dust mite) or ingested (food proteins). Once established, the eczema is self-perpetuating and these allergic components cause no more than worsening of the rash. Removing them, therefore, does not mean that it will disappear.

Atopic eczema usually starts at three to four months of age. It usually appears on the face as a dry, chapped skin or as a teething rash and may spread to cover the body, although it sometimes settles only in the creases of the elbows, knees and neck, when it is called flexural eczema.

Itch is the hallmark of eczema. In the acute phase, little

243

bubbles or blisters are seen in the skin which may break down, weep and crust. Chronic eczema is scaly and dry. It may be so dry that the skin splits or fissures and is extremely painful. Through repeated and prolonged scratching with eczema, the skin may alter in character and look thickened and 'aged'.

People with atopic eczema are prone to skin infections. For instance, they do not cope well with the common cold sore (*herpes simplex* virus). Instead of the infection remaining localised to a small area of skin, it becomes a widespread rash resembling chicken-pox. Bacterial infection is also common, with crusted rashes like impetigo appearing on the skin. Boils also are common. Children who develop eczema early in childhood may develop asthma and hay fever later on.

The outlook for eczema is good and, in most cases, it clears by the age of six or seven years. It may make a brief reappearance around puberty. Some unfortunate individuals do not develop eczema until adult life when it tends to run a much more chronic course.

Treatment

There is no one solution to atopic eczema. Treatment consists of a combination of things. If the person is allergic to inhaled allergens such as house dust mite or pollens, or if there is a definitely established food allergy, every effort must be made to eradicate or minimise exposure to it. But even with doing this, the eczema will need medical treatment. Conventional treatment consists of cortisone (steroid) creams and ointments. These preparations have had a lot of adverse publicity which has done them a disservice because they are extremely useful. Although they can lead to thinning of the skin if over-used, they are invaluable when applied sensibly and under supervision. In the days before they were available, atopic children often became stunted adults because of chronic scratching, lack of sleep and hyperactivity.

Moisturising creams and ointments cannot be over-emphasised as part of eczema treatment. Greasy preparations such as emulsifying ointment BP and Silcock's Base are used in the dry, chronic forms for lubrication and as soap substitutes. Less severe eczema can be moisturised by creams such as aqueous cream BP. When the skin is infected, an antibiotic is needed. Antihistamines may also be useful, especially in helping the sufferer to get a good night's sleep.

Contact dermatitis occurs in two ways. First, repeated exposure to an irritant substance produces a stripping effect on the skin, and dry, chapped eczema appears. Common examples are housewife's dermatitis and apprentice hairdresser's dermatitis, both of which affect the hands. Wet work and detergents, combined with household cleaning agents, are to blame. Anyone who has dry, sensitive skin should be very careful to wear rubber gloves for wet work. If the hands become sweaty, a cotton glove underneath the rubber glove is helpful. People with this type of sensitive skin should use moisturisers regularly.

Allergic contact dermatitis is produced by repeated exposure of the skin to a foreign protein. The most common cause in women is nickel. Nickel dermatitis was called 'suspender dermatitis' in bygone days. The more likely source now comes from jewellery, especially earrings. In men, the most common cause of allergic contact dermatitis is chromate in cement. Other common allergens include hair dyes, rubber, sticky plasters and perfumes. The treatment for contact dermatitis of either sort is first to remove the person from the offending chemical and then to treat as for atopic eczema – with cortisone creams and moisturisers.

PSORIASIS

Psoriasis is one of the common dermatoses or skin diseases. It affects 1 to 3 per cent of the population in this part of the world. Men and women are affected equally. Though it may first appear at any time from early infancy to old age, it usually starts in the teens or twenties. It sometimes appears in response to a sore throat.

The common form is plaque or patch psoriasis. It consists of red, scaly areas which are well demarcated from the normal skin. They are not painful or sore but occasionally itch. The scale is thick and silvery. Common sites are the backs of the elbows, the fronts of the knees and the scalp. The nails are affected with little pits like those in a thimble in 60 per cent of patients. They may also be thickened, yellow and grossly disfigured.

Psoriasis rarely causes ill health but it leads to great psychological suffering from embarrassment. It may give rise to a degree of incapacity although affecting only a small area of skin. For example, severe palm and sole psoriasis may cause great difficulty with walking and working.

Psoriasis is for life and as yet a cure has not been found. It may wax and wane and may even clear altogether of its own accord but it always comes back. It tends to be seasonal, being better in summer than winter.

It is important to realise that psoriasis is neither infectious nor contagious. It is inherited, though not everyone with it has a family history of the disease. In somewhere between 5 and 10 per cent of people with psoriasis, there is an associated joint problem which resembles rheumatoid arthritis. The joints most frequently affected are in the hands, feet and lower back.

Treatment

When it comes to the treatment of psoriasis, time-honoured, non-toxic remedies are still used. Because these treatments are messy, they are best suited to a hospital setting. They include coal tar and dithranol. A course of hospital treatment may lead to a complete clearance of the rash which lasts for up to six months.

Cortisone creams help psoriasis but their place is limited. Their drawback is that psoriasis is a chronic disease that tends to rebound when the cream is discontinued. Also, continued use of strong cortisone cream leads to thinning of the skin. It is important that topical steroids are used only under medical supervision and for limited periods.

A new and very useful ointment containing a vitamin D analogue has recently come on the market. It is called calcipotriol (Dovonex). It suppresses and flattens rather than clears psoriasis but it does not cause a rebound when stopped, nor does it thin the skin. It may, however, cause irritation.

Sunlight is helpful for psoriasis, particularly in people who tan easily. For those with very fair skin, sunburn may occur before achieving a therapeutic dose of ultraviolet (UV). This can make psoriasis worse. Ultraviolet treatment is used in hospital in combination with traditional remedies such as coal tar. It is sometimes used in conjunction with tablets to give a high-intensity form of UV called PUVA. This is effective, but because a high dose of UV is given, repeated courses over many years may lead to skin cancer. For that reason PUVA is used only as a reserve treatment for those with difficult psoriasis.

Though psoriasis rarely causes ill health, there are a couple of forms called erythrodermic and generalised pustular psoriasis that may lead to severe illness. They require hospital admission and urgent treatment. In these cases, very strong oral medication is necessary. This includes methotrexate (MTX), a vitamin A preparation called etretinate (Tigason), or cyclosporin. Occasionally, patients with very crippling or unstable psoriasis may be given these drugs but these treatments are never entered into lightly.

SKIN CANCERS

The Irish are mostly of Celtic races, and so 70 per cent have fair skin that burns easily in the sun and tends to freckle. Skin that burns and does not tan is classified as Type I. In white races, skin types run from I to IV (Mediterranean skin). The lower the skin type, the more prone it is to the toxic effects of sun exposure.

After years of sun exposure, fair skin is susceptible to skin cancer. Those with Celtic skin who live in sunny areas such as Southern Australia are at greater risk than those in their misty country of origin. In Australia, there are excellent educational programmes to alert people to the consequences of sun-worshipping and sunburning. Because the weather in Ireland is often miserable for long periods, people think they are not at risk and throw caution to the wind during a spell of sunny weather. Beware of this, as sunburn predisposes to malignant melanoma. Sunbed UV light is not advisable either. It must be remembered that UV is a form of radiation and that all damage caused by it is irreversible. Sunbed UV contributes to premature ageing of the skin and the development of skin cancers in the same way as natural sunlight does. There is no truth in the story that sunbed tanning toughens up the skin before experiencing the strong sunlight of a foreign holiday.

The most common form of skin cancer is the rodent ulcer or basal cell carcinoma. This appears as a pearly pimple on the skin, usually on the face. It grows in the skin but does not spread to any other part of the body. It gets its name from the fact that it nibbles away at the tissues like a rat. It occurs in both men and women and usually appears in the sixth or seventh decade. It is recently being seen in an earlier age group, presumably due to sunbathing. It is best treated by surgical removal.

The other kind of skin cancer commonly seen is a squamous cell carcinoma. This may follow prolonged sun exposure and also complicates chronic ulcers and sites of irritation such as the lips in pipe smokers. It is a little more common in men. Unlike a rodent ulcer, it may spread via the blood stream or lymphatic system to deposit secondaries in other parts of the body. It is best treated surgically.

Patients developing either of these cancers (referred to as non-melanoma skin cancers) almost always have sun- or photo-damaged skin.

Photo-damage also leads to premature ageing of the skin. The changes due to *anno domini* are called chronological ageing. You can see the difference if you compare the skin on your breasts and buttocks with the exposed skin on your face, neck, backs of hands and front of chest. Photo-ageing produces more changes than chronological ageing and is associated with wrinkling and mottling of the skin. We are all able to tell just by looking at someone whether they have an outdoor occupation, for example, a farmer or a fisherman, or if they have an indoor office job.

From the age of forty or so, in fair individuals who have taken a lot of sun, scaly or warty lesions may appear on light-exposed areas such as the backs of hands and forearms, face and on bald heads. These are unstable areas of skin called solar or actinic keratoses. They are regarded as pre-cancerous. Treatment is by a simple freezing procedure with liquid nitrogen.

We should all be aware that prevention is better than cure and so early avoidance of excessive sun exposure and wearing sunblock creams help to keep the complexion young. There is a lot to be said for the Victorian idea that pale is beautiful.

MALIGNANT MELANOMA

This is the skin cancer that has captured the imagination of the media. While it can occur at any age, it is one that may occur in young people and may have a fatal outcome. To a large extent it is preventable or, at least, detectable at an early stage.

A malignant melanoma arises from the pigment cell in the skin, the melanocyte. About 50 per cent will occur in moles, but the other half arise on what was previously normal skin. There is a definite link between sun exposure and the development of a melanoma. The worldwide incidence of this cancer is increasing at a rate of 10 per cent per year in white people.

There are different types of melanoma. In elderly women, there is a superficial form on the face called a lentigo (freckle-type) maligna. It is flat, large and unevenly pigmented. Though it is slow-growing, it may develop a tumour and therefore should be treated early rather than ignored. A simple procedure, such as freezing with liquid nitrogen, is effective.

In middle-aged adults there is a lumpy type of melanoma called a superficial spreading melanoma. It is two-toned in colour and is flat and raised in different areas. The surrounding skin may be inflamed and it may crust or bleed. Once again, early detection and surgical removal will lead to a complete cure.

The nodular melanoma tends to occur in young people. It is round and raised and varies in size from a few millimetres to, perhaps, a centimetre in diameter. It may occur on any part of the body but if it is on the back it may not be detected until it is too late. It often has a poor outlook by the time it is discovered because the cells are already deep in the skin. The treatment is surgery.

The problem with malignant melanoma is that once it has invaded the deeper part of the skin, it tends to spread through the body by the lymph or blood systems. At this stage, secondary deposits are found in the liver, bones and brain and they are very resistant to chemotherapy and X-ray treatment.

MOLES

Because of the increasing awareness of malignant melanoma, moles are now being viewed as potential time bombs. This, however, is not necessarily so. Only 50 per cent of melanomas arise in moles. It is true that certain moles are unstable and should be checked regularly by a dermatologist but, in general, we should not get neurotic about our moles.

If you have very fair skin which burns easily in sunlight, and if you have over forty moles, it is worth getting them checked. If you have a family history of malignant melanoma you *must* get them checked. If you have twenty or so happy-looking, small round moles don't worry about them – just don't fry them in sunlight. When you are in a very sunny climate, wear a good sunblock.

Please don't start peering at your moles and imagining that some of them are changing. Any change for the worse will be quite definite. However, if you are worried about a mole, an ulcer or any other skin blemish, it it always better to talk to your doctor sooner rather than later.

SUNBLOCKS

Sunblocks or sun screening creams are designed to cut down the amount of UV that reaches the skin. If you have fair skin, it is important to wear them to prevent against wizened, prematurely aged skin. For fair, vulnerable skin, get the highest sun protective factor (SPF) number you can find. The SPF relates to blocking UVB light. Make sure that it is combined with a block for UVA light. Examples of such creams include Sun E45 and Uvistat 30. They will stop you from burning. Read the instructions carefully and make sure to reapply sunblocks if you are swimming. Many of these products are marketed as total sunblocks – but only a thick plank of wood or staying indoors is a complete sunblock!

INFECTIONS AND INFESTATIONS

With better living conditions, better hygiene and better public health awareness, skin infections and infestations are not nearly as common as they were at the beginning of the century. Common infections include impetigo, *herpes simplex* and ringworm.

INFECTIONS

Impetigo

Impetigo is a golden yellow, crusted area on a red background which occurs more frequently in children. It is contagious, ie, spread by touch. It is caused by a bacterium called *Staphylococcus aureus*. Impetigo is easily treated either by an antibiotic cream or, if it covers a wide area, an antibiotic by mouth.

Herpes simplex (cold sore)

This is a contagious viral infection of the skin. Once contracted, the virus will remain dormant in the skin between attacks. These may be precipitated by ill health (colds, pneumonia), sunlight (a sunblock lip balm will help prevent this), stress and other factors. For patients with recurrent *herpes simplex* a cream containing acyclovir (Zovirax), an anti-viral agent, will help to stop an attack.

Herpes zoster (shingles)

This is caused by the chicken-pox virus. People who have had chicken-pox may develop shingles at a later stage in life. It only affects one side of the body and may appear on the head, one limb or on one side of the trunk. The rash is preceded by pain which is sharp because it has a nerve origin. When the rash appears, it consists of red marks with groups of blisters.

Attacks of shingles are more severe in the elderly, who are prone to pain after the eruption has cleared up. This is known as post-herpetic neuralgia. Taking acyclovir in tablet form early in the attack will help to reduce the risk of this unpleasant after-effect.

Ringworm

Ringworm infections are due to fungi called dermatophytes. These organisms are not 'clever' like bacteria, in that they do not become resistant to treatment.

Athlete's foot

Athlete's foot is a very common form of ringworm; the rash may also affect the groins or may appear elsewhere on the body. In the city, the common source of scalp ringworm is cats and dogs, but in the country it is mainly contracted from cattle. Cattle ringworm is particularly nasty, inflammatory and destructive and may lead to baldness if not treated early. Simple forms of ringworm can be treated by anti-fungal creams, but if the infection is persistent, deep-seated or affects hair follicles, an oral anti-fungal drug is given.

INFESTATIONS

Scabies

Scabies is an infestation of the skin due to a mite called an acarus or *Sarcoptes scabeii*. The pregnant female mite burrows into the skin and lays eggs that set off an allergic, itchy reaction in the skin. In adults, itching is from the neck downwards, although it may affect the head in small babies. Scabies is common in conditions of dirt and over-crowding and there is consequently a great social stigma attached to its diagnosis. However, it must be understood that it is endemic (constantly present) in the population and spreads very easily between children. Scabies can occur in the best of families and it is no disgrace! A simple two-night treatment with an anti-scabies lotion such as benzyl benzoate (Ascabiol) will solve the problem. When treating scabies, it is important to treat not only the itchy person but everyone in the household.

Lice

Head lice (*pediculosis capitis*) and body lice (crab lice), sometimes called nits, are also endemic. Outbreaks of head lice in schools do not respect social classes. It is not true that head lice only affect a clean scalp. Again, as in the case of scabies, a simple treatment such as malathion (Prioderm) kills lice effectively. Crab lice respond to the same treatment.

MOISTURISING THE SKIN

Moisturisers and lubricators help to keep water trapped in the skin.

For very dry skin, ointments are best. Ointments are 100 per cent grease. They do not 'go off', as bacteria cannot grow in them. Vaseline is such an ointment. Emulsifying ointment or Silcock's Base are available from the chemist and are equally helpful. The advantage of the last two is that they can also be used as soap substitutes.

Creams are ointments with water added. This cuts down their fat content and allows them to rub in better. They have a cooling effect on the skin and also rub in completely, and so are often called 'vanishing' creams. They suit the average person with slightly dry skin. Because of their water content, preservatives must be added, so creams may potentially irritate.

Lotions have a higher water content than creams. They are useful for removing make-up and provide very little lubrication to the skin.

Dermatology creams which can be purchased over the counter at the chemist shop or sometimes in the supermarket are scientifically tested; it will say on the packaging if preservatives have been added. They contain no perfume. Although many cosmetic firms also produce perfume-free moisturisers, you will pay considerably more for them than for those made by the pharmaceutical industry, including aqueous cream BP or E45 cream.

It is interesting to note that while products produced by the pharmaceutical industry can only be promoted by scientifically established facts, the cosmetic industry may make claims that have no substance to them. For instance, creams containing collagen will not help your skin to look younger in spite of all the blurb on the box. Collagen applied to the skin cannot penetrate it. If it did, it probably would do more harm than good, as it is a foreign protein extracted from calf's placenta. Vitamin E is added to all sorts of creams and lotions but it has no known function. Many creams are marketed with pseudo-scientific jargon and highly coloured diagrams showing how they can bolster out the connective tissue of the skin and reverse wrinkling. None of this is true. If you want to remain young looking like Joan Collins or Elizabeth Taylor at fifty-something, you will have to wear your sunblock all the time, use plenty of moisturiser and have the odd pin and tuck when you begin to sag.

UNWANTED HAIR

It is not true that hair that is shaved or plucked will grow back stronger. Shave, pluck and wax as much as you want. The only way to get rid of hair permanently is by electrolysis. If you are a woman with irregular periods and excess body hair, consult your doctor as you may need to be investigated for a hormone imbalance.

Finally, there is no truth in the rumour that drinking pints of water improves the complexion. It would probably be fair to say that it flushes out the kidneys, but that is as much as you can hope for. Skin is pretty durable stuff. Protect it from UV, give it a little moisturiser when it is dry and it will serve you well.

Dr Sarah Rogers MSc, FRCP, FRCPI is a Consultant Dermatologist and is Medical Director of The City of Dublin Skin and Cancer Hospital, Hume Street.

SLEEP

DR MICHAEL BUCKLEY

Have you ever wondered how your partner can say 'I didn't get a wink of sleep last night!' when you know for a fact that they were fast asleep and snoring all night? Did you know that the average sleeper gets seven hours and forty-five minutes' sleep a night – not quite the eight hours that so many of us crave? Do you sometimes feel cheated because you haven't enjoyed a decent night's sleep in years?

Consultant physician Dr Michael Buckley looks at some of the mysteries of sleep. He explains what happens to us when the lights go out and why we all occasionally have sleeping difficulties.

SLEEP EXPECTATION

Sleep satisfaction, like good health and happiness, is usually only appreciated once it is lost. And like the loss of many valuable possessions, the cause is often carelessness and indifference. To a certain extent, sleep dissatisfaction is related to false expectations. Most adults would have little difficulty in accepting that their sleep requirement in middle age differs from that which they experienced in infancy. However, many middle-aged adults do expect to have the same sleep pattern that they enjoyed in their teenage years, even though they may have no difficulty in recognising (if not accepting) a fall-off in performance in other areas of physical and mental activity.

There is no such thing as normal sleep, just as there is no such thing as normal height, weight, eye or skin colour. We know that healthy people may be tall or thin, black or white, and we know that the range of normality in these people will be very wide and will vary according to age, sex, race and family. We do not expect a two-year-old child to be 1.8 metres tall, to weigh 70 kilos and always to have brown eyes.

In assessing physical normality, we automatically make allowance for a variety of variables, and these allowances must also be made in defining sleep requirement. In addition to age and state of well-being, personality and behavioural factors must be considered. Different people will react differently to similar states, whether these are pleasant or unpleasant. Meat to one person may well be poison to another. Hence, in regard to sleep satisfaction or dissatisfaction, individual reactions come into play which may well be influenced by mood, personality, heredity, environment and, of course, expectation.

THE SLEEP CYCLE

At the beginning of this century, post-mortem examinations of patients who suffered from the now very rare condition known as *encephalitis lethargica* (sleeping sickness) revealed damage to specific areas of the brain which were later found to be involved in the control of wakefulness and sleep. At the end of the first

World War, Hans Berger, an eccentric German psychiatrist, developed a means of recording the electrical activity of the brain on a strip of moving paper – in much the same way as the now more familiar electro-cardiogram records the change in the heart's electrical activity with each beat. Berger's apparatus, the electro-encephalogram (EEG), was first applied to the study of mental illness, but with disappointing results. Shortly before the outbreak of the second World War, American research workers had the novel idea of taking continuous EEG recordings of sleepers throughout the night. They found to their surprise that sleep, far from being a passive process, was one in which a variety of different electrical discharge patterns were emitted from the brain in cycles. Later researchers were to identify rapid eye movements occurring at certain times during sleep, and other periods when these eye movements didn't occur. Sleep was then classified into rapid eye movement (REM) and non-rapid eye movement (NREM) periods.

EEG recordings taken before and during sleep reflect a progressive change in brain-wave pattern. While awake, the waves are small and rapid, but as you pass from drowsy wakefulness to increasingly deep sleep, the wave pattern gradually becomes larger and much slower.

There are four stages of NREM sleep. In stages 1 and 2, you pass from drowsy wakefulness to light sleep; in stages 3 and 4, the deepest sleep is achieved. The first cycle of the night lasts from ninety to one hundred minutes. At that time, about an hour and a half after you go to sleep, just when deep sleep is fully established, there is a sudden lightening or even a short arousal. This is followed immediately by the first and shortest REM period of the night which lasts only a few minutes. The NREM cycle then restarts, this time with a progressive reduction of sleep stages 3 and 4. Thereafter, the night's sleep consists mainly of stage 2 (light sleep) interspersed by four REM periods each lasting ninety to one hundred minutes. The last of these occurs shortly before you wake up.

REM sleep is not classified as either light or deep. It has some of the features of both, but is quite different in other ways. A healthy young adult spends 25 per cent of the night in REM, 20 per cent in stage 3-4 and 50 per cent in stage 2.

Dramatic changes occur during the five REM periods of night-time sleep. The electrical activity of the brain suddenly increases and we dream.

WHAT HAPPENS WHEN WE ARE ASLEEP?

As far as we know, stage 1 sleep is a rather quiet preparatory stage. During it, the protective mental and physical mechanisms against the stresses of the day are gradually toned down in preparation for the further descent that is to follow. Stage 2, on the other hand, is more physically active. This activity takes two forms. First, we change body position every eleven minutes or so. If we didn't, we would develop painful pressure points overnight. The second type of movement occurs when we experience sudden spasms or jerks. These can be forceful enough to wake us up or to disturb our sleeping partner.

When fully established, stage 2 is regarded as the true point of entry into sleep. The interval between lights out and the point at which we reach this stage is termed 'sleep onset latency'. It is a somewhat restless sleep stage. Stage 3-4 sleep is accompanied by a massive release of growth hormone into the blood. The significance of this dramatic and intriguing event is unknown. But we do know that both slow-wave sleep and its growth hormone surge decrease and disappear from the sleep cycle as we get older. It happens to men in middle age and to women a decade later. The hormone testosterone is also released during REM and this can cause penile erections and ejaculations. These are colloquially known as 'wet dreams' and are quite normal.

During REM, breathing is faster and the heart beats more quickly. This is also when most of our dreams happen. We may have pleasant dreams or disturbing nightmares. Nightmares are common in children, especially if the child is unwell or anxious. In adults, nightmares may be a side-effect of certain drugs. How well we remember our dreams depends on the time lapse between REM and when we awake. When someone is awakened immediately at the end of an REM period, they can recall their dreams fully. The longer the arousal is delayed, however, the more fragmented the dream becomes.

SNORING

Snoring is often the source of ribald comment and on occasion the cause of marital disharmony, sibling conflict and death threats from semi-detached neighbours. Occasionally, heavy snoring and grunting are due to a serious condition called sleep apnoea. The sufferer will usually be grossly overweight, have a short thick neck, be a very agitated sleeper and have other physical problems that need medical treatment. Snoring is only one of the symptoms of this condition. By far the vast majority of snorers have no physical problems.

Rhythmic snoring associated with regular breathing is harmless, resulting only in dryness of its perpetrator's mouth. Snorers are often unaware of their efforts and find it impossible to accept that they could make such a noise and still remain asleep. They are not necessarily remarkably heavy sleepers, but as their snoring occurs in deep sleep, they are not easily awakened. During other stages of sleep, snorers are sensitive to other external stimuli, including the snores of their critic at times. Unfortunately, there is no cure for snoring.

RUDE AWAKENINGS, NIGHT TERRORS AND SLEEP-WALKING

Partial arousal from sleep may produce a variety of unpleasant effects, the nature of which is determined by the sleep stage at which it happens. Partial arousals from stage 1 usually occur just as you are going to sleep or immediately preceding the final arousal. In this state, dreams take the form of snapshot impressions rather than the moving picture show associated with REM. These images are invariably frightening and the sense of fear is compounded by an additional sense of immobility and entrapment. However frightening, the episode is short-lived and the person calms down once they are awake.

In certain individuals, particularly in young children, partial arousal occurs in stage 3-4, at the end of the first NREM period and approximately ninety minutes into sleep. Behaviour that accompanies this transition stage includes sleep-walking, night terrors, bed-wetting and teeth grinding. Quite complicated activities can sometimes be undertaken in this state of impaired consciousness. One young patient who was embarrassed by his sleep-walking tried to stop himself by tying his leg to the bed post using a dressing gown cord tied in a series of knots. Ninety minutes or so after sleep onset, he would arise while still apparently asleep and painstakingly untie the knotted cord, free himself, and then proceed to walk ponderously about the house.

There is no treatment for sleep-walking, so it is important to try to make the environment safe, as many sleep-walkers have hurt themselves quite badly, for instance by falling downstairs. Sleep-walking in children usually disappears by the time they are twelve. In adults, it may be a manifestation of stress or conflict.

The night terrors associated with partial arousal from stage 3-4 are different from the flash-point unpleasantness of partial stage 1 arousal. They are longer-lasting (several minutes) and the child may wake up screaming and sweating profusely. They are forgotten the following day. Children usually outgrow night terrors during adolescence.

The most pleasant way in which to wake up is when we have a soft landing resulting from a gradual ascent from stage 2 to 1 and then to wakefulness. When this happens, we wake up relaxed with a feeling of well-being. A bumpy re-entry and hard landing are caused by the sudden intrusion of wakefulness into REM, for example, the ringing of an alarm clock on Monday morning in the final REM period of the night.

HOW MUCH SLEEP DO
WE NEED?

This is like asking how long is a piece of string. Sleep requirement or need, sleep duration and time spent in bed vary from individual to individual. These are all closely related and are subject to both individual and age-related variations. We are all familiar with the 'angelic' infant who sleeps eighteen hours a day and the 'difficult' one who sleeps for only ten. Most people will have come across long and short sleepers. Then there are the 'early birds' and 'night hawks' who go to sleep and wake up at unsociable hours but who sleep the average number of hours.

That there is an average sleep duration is somewhat surprising, in view of the fact that there are so many other variables associated with sleep. Nevertheless, once we reach adulthood – and regardless of age, social background, race, environment and season – the average time spent in sleep is seven hours and forty-five minutes daily. This does not imply continuous sleep, and it is important to remember that when considering elderly people whose bed-time sleep efficiency is impaired by day-time naps. Nor does it imply sleep satisfaction or refer to the quality of sleep.

In middle age, stage 3-4 sleep disappears and it is at this time that the incidence of sleep dissatisfaction and the use of sleeping pills rise dramatically. Sleep dissatisfaction may, of course, occur prior to middle age and may be due to an irregular sleep habit.

SLEEP HYGIENE

From infancy, a basic sleep pattern will be influenced by extraneous factors, particularly by the establishment of a routine, a feeding pattern and a sense of well-being. Later in life, stress, conflict and fear of separation will exert negative influences. Ordinarily, a sleep pattern which is by then established is sufficient to overcome these malign influences, though not necessarily in a single night. Short-term sleep impairment will give rise to short-term sleep deprivation and in turn impose a desire for sleep that will succeed in overcoming the disruptive factors. This introduces the concept of sleep hygiene which is as important to health and well-being as is general hygiene. To take a simple example, regular bowel evacuation can be lost by ignoring the call to defecate at a fixed frequency, which will vary from individual to individual. So too is 'natural sleep' squandered by the loss of routine, whether it is in the infant or the newly 'liberated' teenager. The problem in the early years is that routine cannot be imposed and at times the infant or child might be out of phase with the practice desired by its parents. As in most areas of human activity, a compromise is established, and again as in most areas, common sense wins out and a satisfactory outcome ensues. In the teenager, however, loss of an established sleep pattern is usually due to carelessness: late nights, sleeping until midday when out of school term. It can happen too when people who are unemployed sleep late as there is nothing else to do.

Once the inherent sleeping pattern becomes apparent, we establish it by fixed times and ritual. The toddler who resists going to bed with monotonous nightly regularity is finally brought to bed and will ordinarily sleep within seconds or minutes of completion of an established nocturnal ritual. This usually involves a fixed bed in a fixed bedroom, familiar bed clothes, prayers, teddy bears, a glass of water, stories, lights out – all in the space of minutes and all set against a background of apparent peace and tranquillity. The ritual itself induces sleep and is what the psychiatrists call positive motivation. Any disruption, a different bed or a missing teddy bear, will require significant additional efforts and ingenuity by the carer to reduce the psychological arousal that will keep the child from sleeping. Variations of this ritual apply equally to teenagers, adults and the aged. Those who are fortunate enough to work a five-day week, Monday to Friday, invariably sleep well on Friday and Saturday nights. They experience less satisfaction with their Sunday night sleep, either because of the late Friday and Saturday nights with consequent oversleep on the following days, or because of anticipation of Monday's stress at work.

SLEEP DISSATISFACTION

A poor night's sleep is a universal experience. This may be induced by unaccustomed exercise, mental or physical stress, alcohol, drugs or pain. Frequently, the poor sleeper is told that he or she slept and possibly snored all night. These sorts of isolated episodes probably happen because, although the person apparently sleeps well, they may in fact have entered the light sleep of stage 2 but failed to progress from there to REM, or they may not have had sufficient REM sleep during the night.

Short-lasting sleep difficulties are common when routine is broken – a different bed, a different room, the excitement of travel or the excitement of children on Christmas Eve. When this short-lasting (days to weeks) sleep dissatisfaction occurs, it is called transient situational insomnia. This is a reversible state, but it is imperative that it is recognised and managed in a commonsense manner so it doesn't become a permanent problem.

Sleep dissatisfaction may present in a variety of ways. In whatever way it presents, it must always be regarded as a symptom rather than a diagnosis. The popular image of sleep problems is that they are invariably confined to lack of sleep. This is by no means the case. While there is a general acceptance and apparent understanding for those who complain of lack of sleep, those who sleep too much or who sleep at inappropriate times are slower to discuss their problems. They are afraid people may think they are lazy or even mentally unstable.

INSOMNIA

Insomnia is the mostly widely voiced complaint. This is no more than a symptom, a statement of dissatisfaction. To analyse it further, the type of dissatisfaction must be identified. Do you have difficulty in getting off to sleep (prolonged sleep latency), or maintaining sleep once it is achieved (poor sleep maintenance)? Do you wake up too early (premature final arousal) or, above all, do you feel that you are not refreshed when you wake up in the morning? Once the specific type of complaint is identified, it should be compared to your previous sleep pattern and set against your mental and physical well-being and lifestyle. Obviously, acute and chronic insomnia may occur as a result of pain and a variety of forms of physical distress, for instance fever, or mental illness such as depression, but insomnia can also affect apparently healthy individuals.

The most frequently experienced type of insomnia is termed psycho-physiological. Stress and excitement, whether pleasant or unpleasant, combine to induce a state of both psychological and physical arousal, including mental alertness and an increase in heart rate. The triggering cause is frequently recognised and accepted by the patient, whether it be anxiety, fear, noise, conflict, caffeine, drugs, alcohol, exercise or pre-bedtime activities like chess, bridge or the review of financial affairs, all of which may induce a high degree of mental activity with or without anxiety. When persistent psycho-physiological insomnia occurs, it may have evolved from the transient variety, or its cause may be lost in time. In this situation, the sufferer is in a chronic state of physiological arousal at bedtime and the very ritual of going to bed stimulates further arousal, convincing the sufferer that sleep is impossible over the coming hours.

In the early 1960s, the concept of sleep laboratories emerged in the United States. Initially, insomnia sufferers were investigated in enormously expensive sound-proofed temperature-controlled areas, complete with observation windows, often set in the centre of a working laboratory. This was a highly artificial situation, with the sleep room looking more like an execution chamber than a homely bedroom. Anything less conducive to a satisfying night's sleep could scarcely be imagined! Nevertheless, many of the insomniac patients slept well in these circumstances and often were aware that they had slept well. There are two possible explanations for this apparent contradiction. The first is that some of those who feel they cannot sleep do so, but they are missing the refreshing quality we all associate with sleep. The other possibility is that, removed from the negative motivating factors of their own bedroom and finally receiving the help they had sought for so long, the mental state of pre-bed arousal is reduced. They relax in the knowledge that they are in 'good hands' at last and the resulting sense of tranquillity is followed by sleep.

Other factors that can impede sleep include personality disorders, unrecognised anxiety, depressive states, introduction of stimulant drugs, tolerance to or abrupt withdrawal of sedative drugs, and occasionally disorders such as sleep apnoea.

Those who sleep too much have similar problems and frequently there are quite similar causes. While acute stress, conflict, anxiety or depression will cause insomnia in many, it may cause hypersomnolence (excessive sleepiness) in others which again may be transient or persistent. Similarly, the introduction or withdrawal of drugs may be responsible. It is, however, important to recognise normal variations, in particular in those whose sleep is satisfactory in all respects, other than that it occurs at unsociable times and leaves the individual out of phase with the demands of the society in which he or she lives. In some people, the nightly desire to retire and sleep may be quite fixed, although it may occur much earlier or much later than the time that society considers the norm. As a result, those who wish to retire at six o'clock in the evening and to rise at two o'clock in the morning frequently suffer domestic conflicts and are often referred for 'help'. An even greater problem arises for those who wish to retire at four o'clock in the morning and to rise at noon, and who either report late for work or whose performance is unsatisfactory at work due to sleep deprivation. Others may be contentedly short sleepers or long sleepers, and it would be quite inappropriate in these happy people to attempt to induce 'normal' sleep.

Shift work can also cause sleep disturbance but in general, shift workers seem to tolerate disruption of sleep-wakefulness extremely well. Time-zone transition (jet-lag) can also upset your sleep pattern. The effects vary in intensity from person to person and in the direction of the meridian crossed, for example, it is always worse after flying back to Ireland from the United States than it is when going in the other direction. This type of sleep disruption is usually self-limiting in those who normally sleep well. Problems arise in those who experienced background difficulties prior to the disturbance of their biological clock.

HOW TO GET A BETTER
NIGHT'S SLEEP

There is no magic formula to set right the various forms that sleep dissatisfaction may take in apparently healthy people. The most important rule is prevention. Those who are unaware of a sleep problem are in fact satisfied and they should treat their valuable asset with as much care as they would treat an exotic and expensive possession. For those who are dissatisfied, and where there is no physical disease or mental illness, the best management is usually gained from an understanding of the nature and cause of the problem, accompanied by corrective changes in lifestyle and behaviour.

Where dissatisfaction relates to the quality or the quantity of sleep, there are several practical measures that can be undertaken. It is important to reduce mental and physical activities gradually during the evening. Heavy meals and stimulants such as coffee and alcohol should be avoided before going to bed. Any medication, prescribed or non-prescribed, should be reviewed to determine its potential for disrupting sleep. Those who feel certain that they will not sleep should try to break the negative motivation that has evolved in relation to their bedtime ritual. There is no point in lying in bed for hours, tossing and turning. Time in bed should be significantly curtailed by retiring late and rising early. Initially rest, if not sleep, may well be obtained in a comfortable chair and quiet surroundings. Keeping the time spent in bed short and getting up early at a fixed time will induce sleep deprivation which, in itself, is a powerful stimulant to sleep.

SLEEPING PILLS

Hypnotics (sleeping pills) are recommended by their makers for the short-term management of insomnia. In this respect, they may have a limited role in certain clearly defined clinical situations under strict supervision. Unfortunately, their use and the demand for their use is widespread and the pious recommendations of the pharmaceutical companies are similar to those given by brewers who recommend that a single pint of black liquid is good for you.

The problem arises when a larger volume of black liquid is consumed daily over years. Similarly, long-term use of sleeping pills creates a problem in most but, it must be stated, not in all people. Taken for no more than a week or two, to bring relief in an acute episode of insomnia, the hypnotic may be safely withdrawn once the crisis has passed. Taken for longer, withdrawal becomes more difficult as it is followed by sleep dissatisfaction. If the sleeping tablets are continued, tolerance will develop within some weeks and they will lose their effect. At this stage, the inclination may be either to increase the dose, which restores their effectiveness temporarily, or to withdraw the drug abruptly, which will result at the very least in disrupted sleep. A cyclical situation then occurs, with increasing sleep dissatisfaction resulting from tolerance, loss of efficacy and withdrawal, followed by a day-time hangover effect, either from the drug or from sleep deprivation. Having said this, it must also be said that in some extremely limited circumstances, short-term use of sleeping tablets under guidance may be helpful.

The type of hypnotic prescribed and the nature of sleep dissatisfaction must be carefully assessed. Sleeping tablets vary in the length of time they take to work and how long they work for. A rapid-onset short-acting sleeping tablet may be helpful for someone who has difficulty in getting off to sleep, but it will certainly not be helpful where sleep maintenance or early wakening are problems. Accordingly, when a hypnotic is used, it must be tailored to the type of sleep dissatisfaction for which it is prescribed. Even then, an account of its effect on both physical and mental activities the following day and its cumulative action over several days must be considered if impaired daytime performance is to be avoided.

It must be stressed again that there is no magic in the management of sleep disturbance. Common sense, patience and trust are the most important factors in overcoming a sleep problem.

WHY DO WE SLEEP?

While there is plenty of speculation, virtually nothing is known about the purpose of sleep, despite the fact that about a third of most people's lives are spent in this state. The same question might well be asked of the purpose of the other two thirds of our lives spent in wakefulness, but that is probably best left to the philosophers. Philosophical considerations aside, the purpose of sleep cannot be pursued in isolation but must involve an overview of the sleep-wakefulness cycle.

Some behavioural scientists hold the extreme view that sleep has no function and that it is no more than a habit evolved from early man's desire to while away the hours of cold and darkness when fearful things roamed outside the cave. A trendier view, from what may be called the science fiction lobby, suggests that REM rather than wakefulness is man's prime state.

The middle ground view, based on current knowledge and observation, is rather unexciting if more reasonable. This states that sleep has a restorative function, as yet unidentified, which is necessary for good health.

Dr Michael Buckley MD, FRCPI is Consultant Physician at St James's Hospital, Dublin, and Senior Lecturer in the Department of Pharmacology, Trinity College, Dublin.

SMOKING

CARMEL BUTTIMER

Tobacco is so harmful and so addictive that if cigarettes were invented today, they would surely not be passed as fit for human consumption. Yet cigarettes are seen as a normal part of everyday life. They are available everywhere, even to young children.

ASH Ireland is the new body established jointly by the Irish Cancer Society and the Irish Heart Foundation to lead action on smoking and health in Ireland. Carmel Buttimer is its executive director.

SOME DILEMMAS AND PARADOXES

Tobacco use presents us with a number of dilemmas at both the public policy level and the personal level.

At public policy level, there are ambivalences arising from the paradox of fiscal policy – which provides for the 'health' of the exchequer by means of taxes on tobacco – versus public health policy – which aims to safeguard the health of citizens. This fact immediately questions the logic of whether it makes sense to take in millions from the proceeds of tobacco, only to pay out those same millions in funding the health services which are themselves heavily burdened directly and indirectly as a result of the consumption of that tobacco.

At a personal level, we are now living at a time when there is an unprecedented level of interest and awareness in matters affecting health and lifestyle. The popularity of books on health, dietary preparations, sports equipment and health farm holidays, for example, is evidence of the public concern for health and well-being. The paradox at this personal level lies in the fact that by far the greatest step any smoker can take towards living a long and healthy life is to stop smoking!

Recent years have also brought about an increasing level of concern in relation to the environment and its effects on our well-being. Yet prolonged and consistent exposure to cigarette smoke in one's daily environment presents us with a much more serious and widespread threat than other air pollutants. Independent scientists have estimated that the life-long risk from passive smoking is a hundred times greater than the effect of twenty years' exposure to asbestos in buildings. While these asbestos-contaminated buildings have been evacuated and demolished, a great deal less action has been taken on a product that carries a considerably higher risk.

These dilemmas are carried further into our lives when we shop for food items. Government policy, consumer group action and public concerns in general have contributed positively to the current practice of listing the ingredients on all food packets. Some shoppers even carry a pocket guide on E numbers when they shop. Consumers are demanding food products that are safe and health supporting. Yet what saleable item can rival cigarettes in terms of the hazards involved? This one particular product is responsible for the deaths of one in four long-term users. It should be recalled that the international tobacco industry was aware of the dangers of smoking at least thirty years ago. This information was carefully withheld – the question of public accountability and corporate responsibility clearly did not and still does not arise for the industry. Profit rather than public concern is the order of the day. The health warnings on cigarette packets, the curtailments on advertising and lower tar levels in cigarettes have been imposed by governments, not by the tobacco industry.

It is difficult to understand the willingness of consumers to accept this level of danger in the context of current awareness and concern. It is nearly impossible to imagine a woman buying and using a lipstick, for example, that will convey glamour (and glamour is part of what tobacco advertising promises women) but will endanger the health of her unborn child, and is liable to hasten the onset of menopause. Such a product would undoubtedly be restricted to 'prescription only' access because of its health implications. In the case of tobacco, one consumer in four will die as a result of its regular, daily intake, and yet it is readily available over the counter without a prescription.

The paradoxes and dilemmas in relation to tobacco do not end at the personal and national policy levels. The same ambivalence holds sway in Europe. Tobacco consumption causes close to half a million deaths per year in Europe – a stark statistic. Yet while the European Community contributes £8.5m annually towards cancer prevention, it spends £870m on subsidies to Europe's tobacco growers.

The progress of the very significant EC Directive on the banning of all tobacco advertising has been halted by a small group of four EC national governments due to their own economic interest – either because of their tobacco growers or their tobacco manufacturers. What this adds up to is short-term economics, with little thought given to the longer-term lethal effects of tobacco consumption on the health of nations.

SMOKING WORLDWIDE

The big picture worldwide is now clear. In developed countries, tobacco is currently causing about two million deaths per year, and this number is increasing. Half of those killed by smoking are still only in middle age (ie between thirty-five and sixty-nine). This isolates tobacco use as the most important cause of early death in the developed world.

As the smoking epidemic spreads more extensively to the developing world, tobacco will, in due course, also become a significant killer in those countries. The experience in the developed world clearly shows that this will be only a matter of time.

SMOKING IN IRELAND

The current level of smoking in Ireland is 30 per cent for both sexes over the age of seventeen. While the incidence of smoking among males has reduced steadily from 43 per cent in 1972-3 to 30 per cent in 1991-2, the picture for females is disturbing. There has been no decrease in the number of women smoking in the last fifteen years.

A full half of all deaths in Ireland are caused by just two diseases – heart disease and cancer – and smoking is a major factor in both.

Over 22,000 people die each year in this country from smoking-related illnesses. Of these, there is a core of 7000 deaths that are caused directly by smoking. An important factor to consider among these figures is the incidence of death in middle age as a result of smoking. More than half of all deaths of those aged between thirty-five and sixty-nine are smoking-related. Smoking is therefore the single most significant cause of early death; these people lose an average of about twenty-three years of life. Not only are these years lost, but in many cases, death is preceded by years of illness and debility, as well as by the grief and loss suffered by family, friends and community.

It will be obvious from these figures that tobacco consumption places an inordinate burden on the health services and causes major inroads into the health budget which is funded from the exchequer. Exactly what smoking costs the country is a question of immense consequence for Ireland.

Hospital bed usage is an important indicator, as cancer patients, for example, in some cases may have to stay in hospital for relatively longer periods than other patients. The economic costs of smoking include the industrial costs, such as lower productivity through days lost as a result of sickness, and disability from smoking and passive smoking, including aggravated conditions, as in the case of asthma. It is now known that tobacco is a Class A carcinogen (cancer-causing agent). Smoking in the workplace comprises an important health and safety issue that is only now being recognised in Ireland.

The human costs include the costs associated with some families being thrust into dependency on state welfare as a result of the debility or death of a breadwinner. The costs to the family include the actual cost of buying cigarettes. Smoking in the home also has a heavy impact on children. Passive smoking can be a cause for greater absenteeism from school, greater dependency on family doctors and, in some cases, greater frequency of hospitalisation. There is also evidence of an association between cot deaths and smoking. Additionally, smoking is related to still births and low birth weight.

Quality of life factors should also be included in this assessment. Apart from the loss of years, there is the fact of addiction to consider.

GIVING UP THE SMOKING HABIT

Over 75 per cent of smokers in Ireland would like to give up smoking for both health and cost reasons. For those who want to stop smoking, there is now a great deal of help and advice available in the form of books and other literature, smoking cessation programmes and substitute products. The single most important factor to remember is that, unless disease has already started, it is never too late to stop.

Because nicotine is a drug that causes addiction, it has been described as a 'hellish nightmare' to give it up. Being realistic about this is important. Equally, it is worth remembering that the biochemical agony does not last indefinitely. The addiction itself follows a predictable addiction cycle: a cigarette is needed in the morning for arousal; tolerance develops during the course of the day; and regular doses of nicotine are needed in order to maintain 'normal' functioning.

The essential factor in giving up successfully is personal motivation, coupled with the single-minded determination to beat the addiction. The physical addiction passes quickly for some people; for others it may take longer. Stopping smoking is best understood as a process rather than an event. The process starts with an attitude change wherein the smoker begins to consider stopping. Most smokers know that smoking is bad for their health. But many do not actually know how dangerous smoking is, and many do not know how dramatically risks to health are reduced on quitting.

Next, the smoker should be enabled to translate the resolve to stop into behaviour change, making use of available resources in many cases. For some smokers, will-power alone will be enough. Others will need advice and moral support. Some smokers will find that the ideal combination is will-power, advice and support, and the temporary use of nicotine replacement products. These include nicotine chewing gum, transdermal nicotine patches, and capsules that reduce withdrawal symptoms. Other approaches that are less well researched include cigarette filter solutions, products containing tobacco extract and new nicotine-containing toothpicks.

Withdrawal symptoms are normal. These include elation or light-headedness, irritation, poor concentration, craving, sleep disturbance and short bouts of depression. While craving nicotine, the body is also trying to repair the damage and to adjust itself to change. During withdrawal, you are not only struggling to control the addiction but also missing the 'comfort' of the physical habit of handling and using cigarettes.

It is extremely important for your motivation to remember that the physical withdrawal symptoms peter out in about four to six weeks in most cases. It is also worth assessing your situation fully when planning to stop smoking. Pick a suitable time to begin, perhaps during a relatively stress-free period. For example, women are advised not to stop immediately prior to menstruation.

A plan of action will be of immense help. It should include choosing the day carefully, enlisting the support of family and colleagues, and removing cigarettes, lighters and ashtrays. Think about the sort of situations and occasions on which you usually feel like smoking. Some occasions cannot be avoided, so plan how you will cope in advance. A reward at the end of the first day, one at the end of the first week and another at the end of the first month can help to consolidate your determination to see it through.

Adjustments to the diet are quite important. Vitamin C, especially in the form of yellow fruit, helps the body to rid itself of nicotine more easily and quickly. In the first days of withdrawal, the craving will peak at certain points during the day. This craving peak is unlikely to last more than minutes at a time, so it is sensible to have a ready supply of fruit or orange juice available. Chewing gum (sugar-free) can be helpful at this early stage. Take just one day at a time, one step at a time. Remain positive and determined, taking care not to become complacent by underestimating the strength of the temptation for 'just one cigarette'.

Phase in mild exercise if you have been sedentary. Gradually, this can be increased to light aerobic levels which are well known as 'mood changers' in themselves. This will also increase stamina and maintain metabolic rates at a good level for overall healthy functioning. Exercise further helps to control any tendency towards weight gain. Relaxation techniques are also helpful in counteracting the stresses of withdrawal. Information on these is readily available in books, on tapes and as part of a well-organised smoking cessation programme.

If your first attempt at smoking cessation does not succeed, all is not lost. The reality is that many ex-smokers who have ultimately managed to succeed did so after more than one attempt. A great deal can be learned from earlier attempts to stop, and earlier mistakes can be overcome. So try again. Make sure you really want to stop. Keep a checklist of why you want to stop. The bottom line is to give it up for yourself. Once you achieve this, the other motivating factors will automatically fall into place.

SMOKING AND YOUNG PEOPLE

Eighty per cent of adult smokers in Ireland today had their first cigarette before the age of thirteen, while they were still very much within the education system. By the age of seventeen, one third of all young people are smokers. Of the 55,000 students currently studying for the Leaving Certificate examination, a staggering 18,000 are confirmed smokers. Clearly there is an urgent need for school-based programmes aimed at self-confidence, peer pressure and healthy lifestyles, with a particular emphasis on smoking prevention within an education-for-life curriculum.

Parental influences are the primary determinants of the social and emotional development of the child. The home is the fundamental mediator of social behaviour and sets the basis for the level of the child's self-esteem. For example, peer pressure to begin smoking is better resisted and handled when there is a close connection between parents and children, between parents and teachers, and between the home, the school and the community. If our young people can be enabled to reach the age of nineteen or twenty without smoking, they are far less likely to start smoking at that stage.

Programmes that link health and education at a young age will have effective and lasting results, and in the majority of cases, for life. This is taking responsibility in a genuine and appropriate way for adequately preparing our young people for adult life.

WOMEN AND SMOKING

Women's tobacco use is a serious global issue. Women, and young women in particular, have been identified internationally as a key target group by the tobacco companies. This is reflected in advertising and promotional strategies – images designed to appeal specifically to women; producing new brands for women only, extra-long, super-thin, ultra-low tar, menthol; using other promotions and special offers; and using women's magazines to direct advertising and promotions at women.

In Europe generally, the proportion of smokers in the population has decreased gradually over the last two decades, but the pattern that is now emerging gives significant cause for concern. While for men the decrease has been consistently downward, the consumption of tobacco has increased for women in some countries, notably in France (nearly by half), Germany (75 per cent increase), and Belgium.

There are solid and proven grounds for this concern. In addition to the risk of coronary heart disease, lung cancer and pulmonary diseases, smoking is related to cancers of the larynx, the mouth, the stomach, the bladder and the kidney. Women additionally face the risks of specific gender-related conditions such as cervical cancer, a reduction in fertility, increased risk of ectopic pregnancy and early menopause. The effects of smoking during pregnancy are horrendous. Tobacco poisons cross the placenta to affect the foetus directly. It retards the growth and development of the foetus and therefore reduces infant birth weight. The risks of foetal and neonatal deaths are significantly increased, as are the risks of pre-term delivery and spontaneous abortion.

TOBACCO ADVERTISING

Research undertaken in the USA, Australia and the UK clearly shows that cigarette advertising is a necessary element in the recruitment of children and young people to smoking. Tobacco advertising promotes the idea that smoking is acceptable, particularly when it is associated with sports and other attractive events. The tobacco industry claims that tobacco advertising influences existing smokers only, to either change or maintain brand preferences. However, the adult market is a mature market. Adults who die of smoking-related diseases are not 'replaced' by other adults in maintaining the tobacco market share, since very few people begin smoking in adulthood.

In order to survive in business, the tobacco industry relies on the recruitment of children, teenagers, and in recent years, young women. Children are the future of the industry and are therefore prime targets for tobacco advertising.

The dramatic impact that a total ban on tobacco advertising, sponsorship and other promotion has on consumption of tobacco has been well documented. In Canada, the rate of decline in tobacco consumption has doubled since the ban on advertising was introduced in January 1989. In New Zealand, which introduced its ban in December 1990, there was a reduction in sales of tobacco of over 7 per cent within the first six months, with nearly one in eleven smokers ceasing the habit. The evidence of the impact of advertising bans on consumption is further corroborated by the experience of Norway, with a reduction of 8 per cent, and in Finland with a reduction of 7 per cent.

CLEAN AIR AT WORK

Clinically-clean environments are required for the manufacture of many specialised products. But shouldn't there also be a clean environment for the people working?

The Safety, Health and Welfare at Work Act, 1989 obliges employers in Ireland to provide a clean, healthy and safe environment for all employees. An employer is obliged to draw up a 'safety statement' specifying the manner in which this environment is to be provided. Tobacco smoke in the daily work environment is a Class A carcinogen, in the same category as asbestos, benzene and radon gas. The inhalation of this smoke – known as passive smoking – is damaging to health, particularly in confined areas, and when it happens on a regular or continual basis. In the context of the workplace, the issue is not whether a person chooses to smoke or not. It is a question of where the smoking is done. When a lit cigarette is placed on an ashtray, the unfiltered smoke that enters the air is extremely poisonous, even more so than the smoke exhaled by the smoker.

There is now a ground swell of interest and indeed a growing demand for action in relation to the provision of no-smoking policies in the workplace. A no-smoking policy should act in a positive way for all. For smokers, it identifies clearly where they can smoke, such as the smoking section of the eating area or, if necessary, in a smoking room which has been set aside specifically for this purpose, with its own separate ventilation system. For non-smokers, it removes the health danger and reduces stress among working colleagues. The responsibility for introducing and implementing a no-smoking policy in the workplace lies with the management team. It should be done in a way in which there is genuine consultation with staff, both smokers and non-smokers, and at different levels in the organisation.

PLANNING A SMOKE-FREE FUTURE

Tobacco issues are multi-dimensional. They impinge, either directly or indirectly, on exchequer dependency and taxation, industrial policy, productivity, health economics, education, children, the disadvantaged, health and safety at work, advertising, sponsorship and many more. The issues range from the personal to the collective, from micro to macro levels, from national to global. The solutions must be equally wide-ranging in their scope.

At the personal level, it must be said that smoking is an adult and personal decision and that smoking is acceptable between informed and consenting adults. Anti-smoking initiatives should respect this fact. It is not constructive, helpful or acceptable to cause humiliation or denigration to smokers. For their part, smokers do not have the right to impinge negatively on the health of others through passive smoking, or by example to act as role models, consciously or unconsciously, for children and young people.

Society has a supreme obligation to protect, to educate and to promote the health of all children, and to provide them with the preparation necessary to reach their true potential as adults in society. Children have the right to freedom from tobacco, and this right applies from the pre-natal stage onwards.

The role of legislation in this context is to protect public health and to promote and support policies that are aligned to the implementation of legislation. At the political level, the contradictions between fiscal policy and health policy must be tackled. A planning agenda should be set for the gradual phasing out of exchequer dependency on tobacco taxes, supported by early re-allocation of health funding to embrace a strong and vigorous health promotion and education portfolio. If the incidence of smoking were dramatically reduced, the money saved by individuals would probably be spent on other goods and services, including savings accounts and holidays. These may not carry high tax levels, but in the long term, the exchequer would not be required to sustain current levels to the health sector, since the population would be healthier.

There is a substantial role for industrial policy in relation to tobacco manufacture. Incentives could be made readily available, under certain conditions and within a time-limited framework, to tobacco companies willing to diversify into the production of non-life-threatening products. At social as well as industrial EC policy levels, greater leadership and co-operation is required to tackle the ambivalence and indeed contradictory policies in relation to tobacco growing subsidies on one hand, and health protection and promotion on the other.

National targets should be set for the reduction of tobacco consumption by the years 2000 and 2010, with the means of reaching these targets clearly set out. The dilemmas and paradoxes of tobacco use are compounded by the fact that there are really no technical or scientific obstacles to ending the global smoking problem. Only an integrated set of policies on a range of fronts will effect change in a habit and a custom that has, by default, become endemic. An eminent scientist once said, 'The most dangerous things in the human environment are those that have become comfortable through familiarity.' He was referring to nuclear power plants. Smoking is a pandemic, not unlike a nuclear explosion, but in slow and insidious motion.

Useful address
ASH Ireland, 4 Lr Hatch Street, Dublin 2. Tel. (01) 676 0099.

Carmel Buttimer MSc is Executive Director of ASH Ireland. She has a background in economics, psychology and research and holds a masters degree in social policy and planning.

WEIGHT CONTROL

MARY MOLONEY

One of the best ways to make money these days is to dream up a crazy new diet programme, such as the sausage-and-sodabread diet, or the cucumber-and-custard diet. Give it a catchy title, like 'Flat Bum in Five Days', or 'The D-Plan Diet' (D for daft). Then, sit back and watch your book race up the bestsellers' list. Meanwhile, your grateful readers will probably lose three pounds the first week, six ounces the second week, and by week three they'll be right back where they started.

Crash diets just don't work. But nutritionist dietician Mary Moloney explains that it is possible, and not too difficult, to lose weight permanently – as long as you don't expect miracles overnight . . .

THE SENSIBLE, SUCCESSFUL APPROACH
TO WEIGHT LOSS

According to one dictionary, 'diet' means 'a prescribed course of food devised for medical reasons or as a punishment'. So, by definition, negative connotations are attached to the word 'diet'. With this approach to weight control, the dieter is more often than not doomed to failure. Repeated attempts to lose weight lead to the commonly used term of 'yo-yo' weight fluctuation. The end result is costly, frustrating and possibly injurious to both physical and mental health. To avoid this, a different, positive approach to weight control is necessary. The person should take responsibility for his or her own weight problem and decide to tackle it by:

- sensible eating habits tailored to their own needs;
- some form of regular, moderate exercise;
- changing behaviour where appropriate.

All of these should lead to gradual weight reduction and an increased sense of well-being.

AM I OVERWEIGHT?

Nutritionists and dietitians now use a formula known as the Body Mass Index (BMI) to calculate whether someone is overweight. To get your BMI, divide your weight (in kilos) by your height (in metres) squared. (1 kg=2.2 lbs, 1m=39.3ins.)

$$BMI = Weight (kg) \div Height (m)^2$$

For example, Fiona weighs 62 kg (9.5 st) and is 1.75m (5'8") tall.

$$BMI = 62 \div 1.75^2 = 62 \div 3.06 = 20.26$$

Her BMI is then read from a scale on which different grades are given for different BMI values.

Grade 0	20 — 24.9	Desirable weight
Grade 1	25 — 29.9	Overweight
Grade 2	30 — 39.9	Obese
Grade 3	> 40	Severe obesity

Fiona's BMI of 20.26 falls in grade 0 and indicates that she is at her desirable weight and has no need to diet.

The greater the BMI, the more the individual is susceptible to developing the complications of overweight or obesity. At weights of 60 per cent or more above desirable weight, morbidity (disease) and mortality (death) are approximately double those of the general population.

Overweight is widely recognised as a risk factor for many medical, social and psychological conditions. Medical conditions include heart disease, hypertension (high blood pressure), maturity-onset diabetes mellitus, respiratory distress (breathing difficulties), hiatus hernia (which manifests in heartburn), gall stones, gout (a form of arthritis mainly found in the big toe), and degeneration of weight-bearing joints such as the knees and feet. The overweight body is cumbersome, which in turn causes it to be more accident prone due to lack of agility. Being overweight has also become socially unacceptable. Even at a practical level, severely overweight people are confronted every day by situations that limit their mobility, constrain their social activities and subject them to humiliation – when moving through revolving doors, fitting into seats in waiting rooms, theatres or aeroplanes – not to mention the physical discomfort that is encountered by carrying the excessive weight. Poor self esteem, depression and overeating, sometimes referred to as comfort eating, are all commonly known psychological side-effects of being overweight.

HOW DID I BECOME OVERWEIGHT?

When you take in more energy (calories) than you use, you become overweight. The daily energy requirement varies from person to person. For example, two men, John and Tom, are similar in age, height, occupation and physical activity, but they have very different daily energy requirements. To maintain his body weight, John may have a food/drink intake of 2000 calories. On the other hand, Tom may need a food/drink intake of 2500 calories. Differences in individual energy requirements mean that, on the same daily calorie intake, one person can put on weight while the other maintains his/her normal weight. Overweight people do not necessarily eat more than those who are a desirable weight. However, people who are overweight have at some time consumed more calories from food/drink than they actually require. It follows, then, that a diet that has been specifically designed for losing weight for one person will not necessarily achieve similar results for another person.

The basis for long-term weight control is one of gradual change in eating habits, exercise, attitudes, behaviour and possibly lifestyle.

DIET PILLS

Thousands of pounds are spent each year on books, magazines and special foods or drugs that claim to help weight loss. Dozens of papers are published in scientific journals on the topic each year. Yet the problem persists in our society. It is important to clarify that there is no one miracle drug or food. Over the years, many unsuccessful attempts have been made to manufacture an appropriate drug (anorectic agent) that could promote weight loss. Amphetamines (pep pills) were widely prescribed until their potential for abuse was recognised. Side-effects included euphoria, anxiety and dependence. Withdrawal was found to lead to depression. To date, despite all the scientifically controlled trials, there is no drug available that can make you lose weight without changing your faulty eating habits.

LOW CALORIE LIQUID DIETS

There is no one special food that will promote rapid weight loss. Various low-calorie liquid formula diets are currently being marketed. Most of them provide essential nutrients and high-quality proteins. They come in powdered form and generally contain protein from egg or milk-based sources. This is mixed with water and consumed two to five times a day. They are commonly referred to as 'very-low-calorie diets' or VLCDs. In general, they provide 400-800 calories per day and are designed to produce the largest weight loss possible, while preserving lean body (muscle) mass. It must be emphasised that there are risks associated with their use, as when they are not medically supervised or if they are being consumed by individuals who are not severely overweight, ie greater than 30 per cent of their desirable weight. They are not suitable for someone who is just a stone or so overweight. In mildly overweight individuals, muscle is lost, which in turn can have disastrous consequences, including disturbance in cardiac (heart) function and damage to other organs. The unsupervised use of VLCDs, along with unsuitable dieting, can lead to significant short-term complications such as dehydration, electrolyte imbalance and low blood pressure. Apart altogether from the dangers of using these products, research has shown that the majority of people using VLCDs regain weight almost as quickly as they lose it.

Another slimmers' product now widely available is a liquid replacement meal which comes in various flavours. The theory behind these liquid meals is that they replace the traditional type of meal made from solid foods. Manufacturers state that these meals are nutritionally adequate. However, there are many disadvantages associated with their use. They may be totally inappropriate for individual needs. They are not designed for the user to lose weight permanently. Weight loss may be too rapid, with medical side-effects. They provide no basis for a long-term change in eating habits and are socially unacceptable.

Crash diets – diets that induce rapid weight loss over a very short time – are not recommended either. The reasons are generally similar to those outlined for irresponsible use of VLCDs. Furthermore, they are very often inadequate nutritionally. For example, the banana and milk diet is a poor and unbalanced diet.

The safety of all fad diets is questionable, and they are therefore totally unsuitable for any individual. A comprehensive, long-term weight control programme that is medically recognised is the only effective treatment for overweight that does not have deleterious side-effects.

REALISTIC WEIGHT LOSS

Any weight loss programme must have a multi-disciplinary approach in which the individual takes responsibility for him/herself. First, it is important not to confuse the 'desire' with the 'decision' to lose weight. Decision implies action, whereas desire can be wishful and therefore ineffectual. Once the decision has been made, motivation plays a large role in management. The secret of motivation is self control, which could be defined as running out of excuses not to do the right thing! Factors that can improve motivation include positive support, such as non-food treats from family or friends. Healthy eating for the whole family rather than focusing on one individual has also been found to work successfully on a long-term basis.

A word of caution in relation to 'support'. Nagging a person about his or her weight can be counter-productive and should be avoided at all times. Pressure from society is also best ignored.

A realistic goal for weight loss should be established initially. One pound (0.5 kg) adipose (fatty) tissue in the body is equivalent to 3500 calories, so one must reduce calorie intake and increase calorie (energy) expenditure or physical activity in order to achieve weight loss. For most people, a rate of weight loss of about 1 per cent of body weight per week is appropriate. For example, an adult male with a height of 5'9" (1.75m) whose BMI is 29 and who weighs 14 stone (89kg) should aim to lose two pounds, a little less than 1kg, per week. This moderate weight reduction regime will produce a satisfactory weight loss over a period of twelve weeks without medical or nutritional side-effects. Remember — there is no quick, easy remedy, so patience, a gradual approach and consistency are also important factors to bear in mind. Reliance on restrictive dieting or being in too much of a hurry often end up in 'yo-yo' dieting, resulting in poor self esteem, reduced self control and depression. You shouldn't weigh yourself every day, as daily fluctuations occur. A useful guide is to weigh yourself once a week, with the same clothes on and at the same time of day.

Two national nutritional surveys have been carried out in Ireland, one in 1946 and the other in 1990. Our dietary habits and actual energy (calorie) and nutrient intakes have changed considerably since 1946. The data collected in the 1990 survey, from both children and adults, included BMI, smoking habits, energy and nutrient intake. Of those surveyed, 63 per cent of males and 48 per cent of females were classified as being overweight. In view of this high incidence (which is similar to other populations in the developed world), it is prudent that an overall policy to improve our current diet should be considered.

TACKLING YOUR WEIGHT PROBLEM

• *Plan a management programme.*

At the outset, keep a record in a food diary, documenting the time of day and the quantity of all food and drink consumed. This should span a number of consecutive days, including at least one weekend. The information will give a clearer picture of your dietary pattern and practices. It will highlight the times of the day when possible binge or excessive eating occurs, at night while watching TV, for example.

• *Have a regular meal pattern.*

Never go for long periods without eating. Eat a minimum of three meals per day. Make wise food choices for in-between snacks – they should be low in energy content. Examples include fresh fruit, tea/coffee, water, carbonated drinks that are artificially sweetened, and clear soup. Skipping meals leads to unstructured and consequently erratic eating habits. This scenario leads to 'grazing' or 'nibbling' through the day, resulting in possible intake of excessive energy and food of poor nutritional value.

• *Eat a wide variety of foods.*

Devise a daily meal plan that has a lower calorie content. This ensures that you will have a nutritionally adequate diet.

  *Grill, roast, boil, bake or steam food instead of frying.

  *Use low-fat instead of full-fat products – for example, low-fat spreads, reduced fat milks, low-fat cheeses and yoghurts.

  *Always cut fat off meat.

*Cut down on biscuits, cakes, pastries, chocolates, doughnuts and cream crackers which are all high in fat content.

*Cut down on take-away foods which also have a high fat content – fried fish and chips, fried hamburgers, Indian meals, Chinese meals. Should a situation arise in which the only option for a meal is a Chinese take-away, choose a stir-fry and plain rice in preference to sweet and sour pork and fried rice.

• *Cut down on fats such as cream.*

In general, our diet has a high fat content. Expert scientific committees (the World Health Organisation [WHO], and the American, British and Irish Departments of Health) are unanimous in advocating that all of us, whether overweight or otherwise, should keep down the fat content of our diet. Over the years, several eminent studies have demonstrated that a diet high in fat content is one of the many factors that precipitates the onset of ischaemic heart disease, breast and large bowel cancer and overweight. Gradual reduction of fat intake is recommended.

The goal for daily fat intake should be 30-35 per cent of total calorie intake. A recent American study on women showed that a diet containing 22 per cent fat achieved satisfactory weight loss without having to eat less than they desired. By limiting intake of the foods described, the percentage of energy from fat will remain low no matter what you eat.

Weight from fat is very high (dense) in energy content, eg 1 gramme fat = 9 calories, whereas 1 gramme protein = 4 calories and 1 gramme carbohydrate = 4 calories.

• *Increase carbohydrates.*

The level of carbohydrate foods in our diet is falling. These include bread, cereals, potatoes and pastries. Other sources are sugars, fruits and vegetables, and foods that incorporate these products when manufactured. Current recommendations suggest our intake should be 50-55 per cent of our total energy intake. The 1990 Irish National Nutrition Survey found the actual intake to be in the region of 46-48 per cent.

• *Replace high-fat foods with fresh fruits, vegetables and cereals.*

It is a mistake to think that if you want to lose weight you have to stop eating bread and potatoes. Fibre-rich sources such as wholemeal breads and wholegrain cereals are reasonably low in energy and are preferable to the more refined varieties of bread and cereals. They are fairly inexpensive and should be included in all main meals since they also provide good sources of other nutrients, including protein and some vitamins and minerals. However, should you dislike fibre-rich sources of carbohydrate foods, bear in mind that white bread, refined cereals and pastas also have a high nutritional content – protein, carbohydrate, some fibre and iron – and are major sources of these nutrients in the Irish diet. This can be explained by the fact that, in general, a significant quantity of these foods is consumed on a regular basis, ie at each meal by the majority of the population. Carbohydrate foods form essential components of a sensible eating strategy. As part of a weight loss plan, it is advisable to reduce overall daily intake of these foods by approximately 25 per cent.

Fruits and vegetables (all varieties of both) are less dense in carbohydrate content than breads and cereals. They are useful, palatable foods which can be easily incorporated into the diet two to three times daily. They provide vitamins, especially folic acid, vitamin C and some minerals. Citrus fruits and the coloured vegetables, including dark green cabbage, broccoli, carrots and peppers, have the highest concentration of these vitamins. The vitamins are easily destroyed by excessive boiling or by the addition of bread soda to the cooking water. Fresh (provided it is genuinely fresh) and frozen varieties have the highest nutritional content. Tinned fruits and vegetables have limited quantities of vitamin C. Pulse vegetables such as peas, beans and lentils are useful, inexpensive sources of protein, carbohydrate and consequently energy.

• *Cut down on sugars.*
Sugar in various forms, including puddings, meringues and jams, may contribute to the development of overweight/obesity. Omission of sugars from the diet, though safe, is not usually sufficient as a weight-reducing regimen. Sugar foods are known to be energy-dense and are rarely high in vitamin or mineral content. Consequently, they are not on the 'recommended' list of

291

foods to be encouraged when tackling a weight problem. As a person gets into the habit of eating low-fat, low-sugar foods, and eating three meals each day, the desire to binge-eat will diminish. Cravings for high-sugar foods should become less frequent and so eating any of them will fall into the 'normal' category. If you get the urge to consume these foods, limit the quantity, or better still, eat fresh fruit as a substitute.

Always remember the saying: 'If at first you don't succeed, try, try again.' Never, never give up in desperation. Just because you make a slip and give in to the craving for a bar of chocolate, there is no need to abandon all the days and weeks of effort. One or two lapses won't undo all your good work.

Alcohol also has a high energy content and has little other nutritional value. One gramme of pure alcohol yields seven calories. A pint of beer has 160 calories, a gin and tonic has 158, and a glass of wine has 90. If you are serious about losing weight, alcohol should be reserved for the celebratory drink when you have reached a realistic target weight.

• *Get some exercise!*
Exercise in moderation is strongly encouraged. Psychologically, it provides a feeling of well-being and helps to take the mind off food. Check with your GP before starting an exercise plan. Begin slowly and gradually increase the duration and intensity. For example, commence by walking for ten to fifteen minutes per day. As you become accustomed to longer walks, quicken the pace while making sure it is not too strenuous. If you are still excessively tired an hour or two after walking, the walk was too strenuous. Next time, reduce the pace and the distance.

Other forms of exercise that can easily be undertaken in the normal daily routine include taking the stairs instead of the lift, getting off the bus a few stops before or after your usual stop, or doing some outstanding household chore instead of watching television! Swimming, cycling, playing tennis or golf, or gardening regularly are other sensible forms of exercise. Without a change in dietary habits, exercise will achieve little if any weight loss. The aim is to combine an eating plan that has a lower energy value than the 'usual' food consumed with a regular moderate exercise plan.

• *Develop good eating habits.*

Good eating habits do not start at the table, but in the supermarket. Useful tips include making a shopping list and sticking to it, never shopping when you're hungry, avoiding ready-made meals and take-aways, and carrying only the cash you need for the food on your list.

Throughout the day, try to eat meals and snacks at scheduled times. Do not skip meals. Don't eat while doing something else. For example, don't have coffee and biscuits while you work, and don't munch your way through a bag of crisps while watching television. Substitute exercise for snacking. Stick to your eating plan. If someone offers you food, don't accept it.

At mealtimes, chew food thoroughly and eat slowly. Should you wish to have second helpings, choose wisely – for example, vegetables or fresh fruit. Leave the table as soon as you've finished eating. If there is an invitation to a party, try to drink bottled water, low-sugar drinks, tea or coffee. Reduce alcohol consumption to a minimum or alternate it with bottled water. It may be helpful to take a low-energy snack beforehand, such as a low-fat yoghurt, in order to avoid overeating late in the evening.

It is wise to reduce excessive body weight when it impairs your quality of life and threatens your medical, physical, social and psychological well-being. Changing attitude or behaviour in relation to dietary habits can be a slow process. However, it is achieveable, since the responsibility mainly lies in your own hands. Safe, permanent weight loss cannot be achieved quickly. Strategic planning in changing your pattern of food intake, exercise and behaviour are essential. If you have personal commitment and patience, you'll find this programme does work.

Dr Mary Moloney Dip Diet, MSc is Senior Lecturer in Human Nutrition and Dietetics at the Dublin Institute of Technology, Kevin Street.

APPENDIX

INCIDENCE OF BREAST CANCER

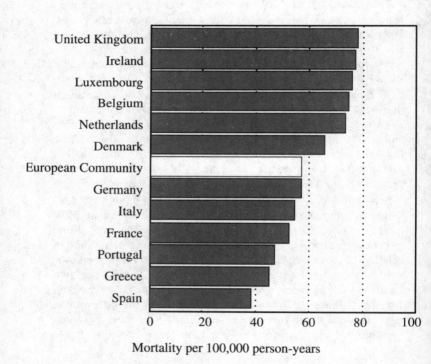

Mortality per 100,000 person-years

RECOMMENDED READING

Brady, T. 'Paradoxes in the Pursuit of Psychological Well-Being', *The Irish Journal of Psychology,* 11, 3. The Psychological Society of Ireland, Dublin, 1990

Carson, Dr Paul. *How to Cope with Your Child's Allergies* and *Coping Successfully with Your Child's Asthma.* Sheldon Press, London

Comfort, Alex (MB, PhD). *The Joy of Sex.* Quartet Books, London

Coni, N, Davison, W and Webster, S. *Ageing: The Facts.* Oxford University Press, 1992

Dalton, Katherine. *Once a Month.* Fontana, London

Duckworth, Helen. *Premenstrual Syndrome, Your Options.* Attic Handbooks

Gayson, M I V. *Back Pain — The Facts.* Oxford University Press

Gillett, R. *Overcoming Depression.* Dorling Kindersley, London, 1987

Harrison, Dr Michele. *Self-help with PMS.* Optima

Hartman, Ernest. *The Sleeping Pill.* Yale University Press, 1978

Kenzie, Robin M. *Treat Your Own Back.* Spinal Publications Ltd

Kushner, H. *Why Bad Things Happen to Good People.* Tavistock Publications, London, 1982.

Lewis, C S. *A Grief Observed.* Faber & Faber, London, 1961

Morrow Brown, Dr H. *The Allergy and Asthma Reference Book.* Harper & Row, London

Oswald, Ian & Kirstine, Adam. *Get a Better Night's Sleep.* Martin Dunitz Ltd, London, 1983

Parkes, C M. *Bereavement Studies of Grief in Adult Life.* Tavistock Publications, London, 1972

Royal College of Psychiatrists (1986). *Alcohol: Our Favourite Drug.* Tavistock Publications, London

Rush, J. *Beating Depression.* Century Publishing, London, 1983

Sherwood, Dr Paul. *The Back and Beyond.* Arrow Books Ltd, London

Shreeve, Dr Caroline. *The Premenstrual Syndrome.* Thorsons, London

Stewart, Maryon. *Beat PMT Through Diet.* Edbury Press

Stroebe, W & Stroebe, M S. *Bereavement and Health. The Psychological and Physical Consequences of Partner Loss.* Cambridge University Press, Cambridge, 1987.

Unsworth, Heather. *Coping with Rheumatoid Arthritis.* W & R Chambers Ltd, University Press, Cambridge

Wainwright, Denys. *Arthritis and Rheumatism.* Paper Fronts, Elliots Rightway Books.

INDEX

A

acne vulgaris, 240-3
acupuncture, 56
adolescence
 and PMS, 215
ageing. *See* growing old
AIDS, 237-8
 and the dentist, 192-3
alcohol, 9-21
 abuse of, 10
 and the Irish, 10-12
 alcoholism, 12-14
 safe drinking, 14-15
 and women, 15-16
 detection of problems, 16-18
 treatment of abuse, 18-20
 and young people, 20-1
allergies, 23-34
 definition of, 24
 signs of, 24-5
 causes of, 25-6
 most common conditions, 26-8
 starting age, 28-9
 food allergies, 29-31
 testing for, 31-2
 treatment of, 32-3
Alzheimer's disease, 127-8
ankylosing spondylitis, 38-9
arthritis, 35-43
 types of, 36-40
 risk factors, 40-1
 prevention, 41
 exercise, 41-2
 future treatments, 42
 management of, 42
asthma, 26, 27, 104-7

 treatment of, 106
athlete's foot, 252

B

back pain, 45-60
 causes of, 47-8
 diagnosis of, 48-9
 prevention of, 49-52
 body mechanics for lifting, 52
 factors contributing to, 53
 treatment of, 53-9
 spinal surgery, 59
 keeping in good condition,
  59-60
bereavement, 61-76
 reactions to loss, 63-4
 protective phase, 64
 confronting the loss, 64-7
 learning to live with loss, 67-8
 nature and circumstances of,
  68-9
 characteristics of bereaved
  69-71
 consequences of loss, 71-3
 helping the bereaved, 73-5
blood pressure, 125-6, 139
bone, ageing of, 125
bowel problems, 77-85
 bowel conditions, 78-84
 dietary fibre, 84
 bowel tests, 85
 danger signals, 85
breast cancer, 87-98
 risk factors, 89
 breast pain, 89-90
 detection of, 90

self-examination, 90-1
signs and symptoms, 91
mammography, 91-2
treatment of, 92-3
surgery, 93
breast reconstruction, 94-5
radiotherapy, 95
chemotherapy, 96
hormonal therapy, 96-7
long-term outlook, 98

C
CAGE questionnaire, 16-17
cancer
bowel, 82-3
breast, 87-98
prostate, 168-70
testicular, 172
oral, 190
skin, 247-50
candidiasis, 235-6
cardiovascular disease, 177-8
cataracts, 124
chemotherapy, 96
chiropractic, 56
chlamydia trachomatis, 231-2
cold sores, 188-9
colitis, 80-1
connective tissue disorders, 39
constipation, 83-4
coughs, 99-107
definition of, 100-2
medical approach to, 102-3
wheezes, 103-7
crab lice, 253
Crohn's Disease, 80

D
dentist
and HIV infection, 192-3
you and the, 193-4
fear of, 194
depressive illness, 109-17

symptoms of, 110-12
prevalence of, 112
causes of, 112-14
treatment of, 114-16
outcome of, 116
prevention of, 116-17
dermatitis, 243-5
desire, lack of, 225
diet
and heart disease, 133-8
and PMS, 214-15
diverticular disease, 81-2
dyspareunia, 223
dyspepsia, 146

E
eczema, 27-8, 243-5
ejaculation, problems with, 224-4
electro-convulsive treatment
(ECT), 115
electrotherapy, 55
erectile difficulties, 224
eyesight. See vision

F
fertility. See infertility
fluoride, 186

G
gastroenteritis, 79
gate-control theory, 197-9
genital warts, 234-5
glaucoma, 123-4
gonorrhoea, 230-1
gout, 39
growing old, 119-29
life expectancy, 120-1
misconceptions, 121-2
and modern medicine, 122-3
skin, 123
vision, 123-4
hearing problems, 124-5
bone and muscle, 125

blood pressure, 125-6
intelligence and memory, 126-7
exercise, 127
early identification of problems, 127-8
in society, 128-9
gum disease, 183-4
gum recession, 185

H
haemorrhoids, 79-80
head lice, 252
hearing
and ageing, 124-5
heart disease, 131-44
symptoms and signs, 132-4
causes, 133
and diet, 133-8
smoking, 138-9
risk factors, 138-40
family history, 139-40
investigating, 140-1
treatment and recovery, 141
community action, 141-2
glossary of terms, 142-3
heartburn, 146-9
hepatitis B, 236-7
herpes simplex, 188-9, 232-4, 251
herpes zoster, 251
HIV, 237-8
HIV infection
and the dentist, 192-3
hormonal therapy, 96-7
Hormone Replacement Therapy (HRT), 178-80
hormone therapy, 216-17
hydrotherapy, 57
hyperactivity, 31

I
impetigo, 251
impotence, 170-1
in vitro fertilisation (IVF), 162-3

incontinence, 83
indigestion, 145-9
investigation of, 147-8
treatment, 148-9
complications, 149
infertility, 153-63
causes of, 154-6
testing for, 156-9
treatment, 159-61
new technologies, 161-2
test-tube babies, 162-3
insomnia, 263-5
irritable bowel syndrome, 78-9
isometric exercises, 57
isotonic exercises, 57

L
lice, 253
life expectancy, 120-1

M
mammography, 91-2
manipulation, 55-6
massage, 54
melanoma, malignant, 244-5
menopause, the, 173-80
reasons for, 174
symptoms of, 174-5
backdrop to, 175
features of, 175-7
osteoporosis, 177
cardiovascular disease, 177-8
Hormone Replacement Therapy (HRT), 178-80
diet, exercise, recreation, 180
and PMS, 216
men's problems, 165-72
prostatism, 166-8
prostate cancer, 168-70
impotence, 170-1
testicular cancer, 172
sexual problems, 224-5

mercury
  in amalgam, 191-2
moles, 250
mouth and teeth, 181-94
  common diseases, 182-3
  hygiene and prevention, 184-5
  gum recession, 185
  fluoride, 186
  orthodontics, 186
  dentures, 186-7
  pain and toothache, 187-8
  discoloured teeth, 188
  cold sores and herpes simplex,
    188-9
  mouth ulcers, 189
  impacted wisdom teeth, 190
  oral cancer, 190
  crowns and bridges, 190-1
  implants, 191
  mercury in amalgam, 191-2
  HIV infection and the dentist,
    192-3
  you and your dentist, 193-4
  fear of dentist, 194
mouth ulcers, 189-90
muscle, ageing of, 125

N
night terrors, 260

O
oral cancer, 190
orgasmic difficulties, 223-4
orthodontics, 186
osteoarthritis, 36-7, 125
osteopathy, 56
osteoporosis, 125, 177

P
pain, 195-206
  types of, 196-7
  gate-control theory, 197-9
  communication of, 199-200
  relief and management of, 200-4
  pain-killers, 201
  patient-controlled analgesia, 202
  psychological approaches, 202-4
  in terminal illness, 204-5
  relaxation techniques, 205-6
periods. See premenstrual
syndrome
piles, 79-80
plaque, 182-4
PMS. See premenstrual syndrome
polyps, 82
premenstrual syndrome, 207-18
  definition of, 208
  sufferers from, 208-9
  causes, 209
  symptoms, 209-10
  diagnosis of, 210-11
  unsympathetic doctors, 211-12
  self-help, 212-14
  and diet, 214-15
  adolescence, 215
  exercise, 215
  and menopause, 216
  medical treatments, 216-18
  final choices, 217-18
prostate cancer, 168-70
prostatism, 166
  treatment of, 166-8
psoriasis, 245-7
psoriatic arthritis, 39
psychotherapy
  depressive illness, 115-16

R
radiotherapy, 95
reflexology, 56
relaxation techniques, 205-6
rheumatism, 40
rheumatoid arthritis, 37-8
ringworm, 251

S

scabies, 252
sex therapy, 225-8
sexual difficulties, 219-28
  sex and sexuality, 220-2
  sexual problems, 222-5
  treatment, 225-8
  sources of help, 228
sexually transmitted diseases
    (STDs), 229-38
  definition of, 230
  gonorrhoea, 230-1
  chlamydia trachomitis, 231-2
  herpes simplex, 232-4
  genital warts, 234-5
  trichomoniasis, 235
  thrush (candidiasis), 235-6
  hepatitis B, 236-7
  HIV and AIDS, 237-8
shingles, 251-2
skin, ageing of, 123
skin problems, 239-54
  function of skin, 240
  acne vulgaris, 240-3
  eczema/dermatitis, 243-5
  psoriasis, 245-7
  cancers, 247-50
  moles, 250
  sunblocks, 251
  infections and infestations,
    251-3
  moisturising, 253-4
  unwanted hair, 254
sleep, 255-68
  expectation, 256
  sleep cycle, 256-8
  what happens during sleep,
    258-9
  partial arousal, sleep-walking,
    259-60
  snoring, 259-60
  amount of sleep needed, 260-1
  sleep hygiene, 261-2

  sleep dissatisfaction, 262-3
  insomnia, 263-5
  how to improve, 266
  sleeping pills, 266-7
  reasons for, 267-8
  sleep-walking, 260
smoking, 269-81
  and heart disease, 138-9
  and the menopause, 180
  dilemmas and paradoxes, 270-2
  in Ireland, 272-3
  giving up, 273-6
  and young people, 276
  and women, 277
  tobacco advertising, 277-8
  clean air at work, 278-9
  planning smoke-free future,
    279-81
snoring, 259
STDs. *See* sexually transmitted
    diseases
stomas, 84
stress, 139
sunblocks, 251

T

teeth and mouth, 181-94
  hygiene and prevention, 184-5
  toothache, 187-8
  discoloured teeth, 188
  impacted wisdom teeth, 190
  you and your dentist, 193-4
  fear of dentist, 194
terminal illness
  pain in, 204-5
test-tube babies, 162-3
testicular cancer, 172
thrush, 235-6
traction, 55
trichomoniasis, 235

U
ulcerative colitis, 80-1
ulcers, 145, 149-52
  diagnosis, 151
  treatment, 151
  medication, 152
  surgery, 152
urology, 165-72
urticaria, 28

V
vaginismus, 223
vision
  and ageing, 123-4

W
weight control, 283-94
  sensible approach to, 284
  calculation of overweight, 284-5
  reasons for being overweight,
    285-6
  diet pills, 286
  low calorie liquid diets, 286-7
  realistic weight loss, 288-9
  tackling the problem, 289-93
wheezes, 103-7